How to Reduce Your Weight

How to Reduce Your Weight

Cross land
BOOKS

HOW TO REDUCE YOUR WEIGHT
ISBN 81-8408-135-9

First Edition : 2008

Published by :
INDIANA PUBLISHING HOUSE

For

Crossland BOOKS

2/13 Ansari Road, Darya Ganj,
New Delhi-110 002

Printed by:
Salasar Imaging Systems
C7/5, Lawrance Road Indl. Area, Delhi 110 035

Contents

Why Not You?

Excess weight is a misfortune that can become a real mental burden to those afflicted with it. Even if the problem does not necessarily represent a danger to physical health, its psychological effect alone can be serious matter.

The medical profession sometimes seems uninterested in overweight, unless it is so far advanced as to constitute obesity.

It is doubtful that the problem of excess weight arouses enough concern, especially in view of its potential dangers.

Excess weight should not be regarded simply as a misfortune. The problem calls for medical attention—not only on account of any mental distress it may entail but because it can possibly, in spite of its appearance of well being, represent the first stage of a serious affliction.

People who are "well-built" (really meaning "plump") want to know why they are as they are, just what mechanism is causing it, whether it can be easily cured, if it is serious and, above all, what they must do to recover their figure!

In this book, the very latest discoveries and treatments for this problem are discussed.

There has been so much said about overweight, and so much nonsense talked, that there is a real need for a summary of whole subject that is theoretical enough to be interesting, practical enough to be effective and, especially, clear enough to be understood.

Everyone to-day knows that 90% of the fat men and women can and should slim under doctor's orders and without affecting their health, this can be achieved without either pain or magic. Anyone can, with will-power and patience, slim without tears!

Chapter I

What Causes Overweight?

At last it's all over! The glands myth, very fashionable since 1930, has gone overboard and now almost the entire scientific world is in agreement. The old endocrinology theory on excess weight seems to be fading out.

Endocrine forms of obesity do undoubtedly exist. These cases are quite clear and well-defined, and represent *no more than one or two per cent of all cases of obesity.* They are of too scientific and speculative a character to be dealt with in a practical book for popular consumption.

THE NERVOUS CENTRES OF OVERWEIGHTS

The "Junction!"

It is indisputable that, if you eat properly, you are unlikely to get fat.

It is now agreed that there is a *reserve distribution centre in our organism,* no doubt hidden away in some corner of the brain that controls the accumulation and balance of the fat in our bodies.

Any lack of balance in this centre is clearly of prime importance, since not only do we see two people who are following the same diet putting on weight unequally, but, more particularly, the same person's weight can change suddenly without his or her eating habits having changed a jot.

Although we are still only at the hypothesis stage, a whole series of facts leads us to suppose that this central mechanism is situated between and below the cerebral hemispheres, behind the pituitary gland, in what is called the floor of the third ventricle of the brain or the "hypothalamus." Anatomically, this centre is situated in the diencephalic region which forms parts of the "central nervous system," that is, of the brain.

There is an important and curious coincidence. This "diencephalic" central distributor of the connective tissue, watery or fatty, is also the centre of our emotional life. Moreover, this important junction, this centre of our emotional life, is directly related to:

- The whole of the sympathetic and para-sympathetic nervous systems.
- The whole of our internal gland secretion system. These three (diencephalic-sympathetic-glandular) seem to form an inseparable whole, a "trio" which truly controls the operation of the human machine.

In this book, not to be over-technical, we shall call this region "the junction."

Nervous Overweight

Now that we have located this central regulatory factor on which the metabolism of fats and water would seem to depend, lets us see how this centre imposes its will. But let us first define the word "metabolism." It means simply the process, within our bodies, by which nutritive material is built up into living matter.

It is believed that it is the sympathetic nervous system which transmits orders from the junction and that it is, along with the endocrine system, itself part of the junction.

We can often clearly see the part played by the sympathetic system in cases of "nervous obesity." Everything happens as if, at a given moment, the sympathetic fibres, which simply should pass on the junction's orders, get out of hand and reinforce the orders received from the central authority too strongly. These are cases of sympathicotony, or an exaggerated toning up of the sympathetic system.

Sympathicotonic obesity is usually accompanied by other upsets. Actually, although the sympathetic system plays a part in storing fats, this is far from being its only function. The whole of our cardiovascular and mental functioning, as well as that of our internal organs, etc., is governed by the nervous system, in balance with its opponent, the parasympathetic (or pneumogastric) system.

As the vitality of the sympathetic system seems to favour the accumulation of fat we can readily understand that signs of hypersympathicotony, such as hypertension, intestinal sluggishness, and dryness of the mouth, accompany overweight. On the other hand, it is clear that if the sympathetic system becomes inadequate and allows itself to be supplanted by its opponent, the pneumogastric system, the result is loss of weight accompanied by low blood pressure, spasms of internal organs, nervous depression and nausea.

The sympathetic and the pneumogastric systems are like two rivals who are continually fighting each other. The one is miserly and the other spendthrift. It depends on which has the ascendancy, when there is extreme parsimony, the result is overweight. When there is a wild spending, thinness results.

Overweight Classified

In this book, we shall divide overweight into three categories: fatty overweight, watery overweight (or spongy overweight) and cellulitis. These three categories are very different as regards their appearance, mechanism and treatment. But these categories can overlap and mix, anyone of the three predominating in varying proportions.

Fatty overweight is really "fat and muscle" hypertrophy (excessive growth). It is uniformly spread, is accompanied by a large appetite and is more usual in men.

Watery overweight is a matter of "watery fat." It doesn't affect the muscles at all, it is most usual over the lower half of the body, is not accompanied by any marked appetite, and is most common in women.

Cellulitis is a form of infiltration rather than overweight.

Chapter II

Fat in the Body

FAT IS AN UNWELCOME VISITOR

There is always fat in our body. It is only when there is too much of it that we are entitled to talk of being overweight. It acts at the same time as a storeroom for our bodies and as a protective cushion.

Fat makes a covering on the surface of our bodies. It is about a quarter of an inch thick under the lower layer of the skin, where it fills the gaps in the cellular spaces or subcutaneous tissue. It gives the skin its appearance of fullness, and ensures suppleness of the body's movements. It is thickest in certain places where, in some overweight people, it forms veritable rolls of fat, usually on the stomach, the breasts, the thighs, hips and the buttocks. In the normal body, the layer at these places should be no more than a half-inch-thick. If the person is overweight, the fat spreads everywhere, but will be at its maximum in these areas.

Fat surrounds many of our organs. It is around the

heart, for instance. Where there is overweight, it accumulates there to such an extent that it may compress it, hinder its movements and cause pain. It will weaken this organ all the more when, as so often happens, it doesn't just hinder its movements, but infiltrates it and reduces its muscular strength.

Fat is especially found in the *stomach* and in the peritoneum, where numerous folds protect our abdominal organs and bring them what they need to function. Some may, however, develop into a layer of fat (epiploic fold).

The *kidneys* are also surrounded (within the sac in which they are contained) by a cushion of fat which protects them against prolapsis or rupture, a not uncommon occurrence in thin people.

On the other hand, fat is rarely found around the lungs, the brain, the genital organs and the spleen.

Fat in general, apart from the aesthetic objections and the troubles, and illnesses to which it can give rise, has the grave disadvantages of making surgical operations (and particularly abdominal surgery) very difficult.

Your Body is a Laboratory

Chemically, the fat in the body can come from the fat we eat. But the body is a sufficiently powerful biochemical laboratory to be able to manufacture fat simply out of carbon, oxygen and hydrogen, which are its basic components. We get these same components when fats are broken down or burned. Carbonic acid and water, which are the normal residues when fats are broken down, are carbon, oxygen and hydrogen.

Now it can be seen why it is not even necessary to consume fatty foods, whether vegetable or animal, to become fat; sugar lean meat and lentils, among other things, can be sufficient raw material for that marvellous factory which is our body. So with a person whose stoutness results from food, cutting out fat won't suffice. He must restrict his diet beyond this.

We are forced to another conclusion: that water, which is made up of oxygen and hydrogen, possesses in itself two of the three elements required for making fat. This fact has for a long time shown the importance of water in overweight, and we know that more than half the cases of corpulence are due to water.

Where Does Fat Go?

Fat consumed, which represents a large part of the fat stored by the body undergoes chemical changes in the intestines before passing into the blood.

If the fat is not used up right away as fuel needed by the body (for a work load or, for example, exercise, etc.) it becomes over-concentrated in the blood and the blood unloads it into the connective tissue. It then becomes a reserve of dormant fat.

On the other hand, when blood has used up too much of it, it will then find itself somewhat short of fat. It will draw reserves from the connective tissues and carry them in its stream for use when needed. When this happens, it decomposes the fatty particles by combustion, and the residue is water and carbonic acid.

Fat is Our Fuel

Fat is the best fuel for the machine which is our body. It is the material whose combustion produces the most heat (this combustion in our bodies is simply a slow oxidation). Every ounce of the fat produces some 250 calories. Naturally, the colder the country we live in, the more fat we have to make.

Our system maintains our body temperature by burning up the fats it has in reserve. The colder the air, the more we need. All animals living in the cold countries have been provided by nature with a thick layer of fat.

Chapter III

Watch Your Weight!

LOOK OUT FOR TROUBLE!

Before trying to define overweight, it seems sensible to define the conventional standards of normal bodily sizes, weights and shapes so that the men and women who read this book may know how far they are from the ideal. The table of measurements we have prepared for women (see the end of the book) will give them more precise information on this subject. But let it be clear now that those who undertake a course of treatment must weigh themselves regularly every month, at the same time of day (the same day of each menstrual cycle for women).

Women try to get their figure back for the sake of their appearance, and they are right. It is only too obvious that getting fat means looking older, losing your charm, spoiling the style of your well-cut dress. It also puts them at a disadvantage socially and in business. The more attractive a saleswomen or an interviewer looks, the more persuasive she will be. The same arguments apply to men.

Getting fat is neither a normal development nor a privilege of age. It begins the departure of youth, and not only of youthful appearance, it means loss of enthusiasm, of the joy of living, of versatility, of physical and mental vigour. It brings short-temper, tiredness, loss of memory, drowsiness, digestive upsets and nervous instability.

Here is something to think about. We have now gone beyond the stage of beauty pure and simple. Watch out! A successful marriage demands daily renewal. Don't rest on your laurels. See the danger from the start and put things right without delay.

YOUR IDEAL WEIGHT

According to an old conventional standard a man should weigh 5½ times as many pounds as he is inches taller than 3 feet 3 inches. For example: 5 feet 7 inches = 154 pounds. Actually, this rule works only for people of middle height and gives an excessive result by about 10 pounds. It works reasonably however, for a man who is fully clothed. A man fully dressed, 5 feet 7 inches tall, should weigh approximately 154 pounds.

This method of calculation is in any event too high for a woman. Her weight proportions are different from those of a man. Her muscular development is considerably less. It reaches only 36% of her weight, whilst for a man it is 50%. This is all the more important since the muscles are the heaviest component of the body, after the bones. We must realize too that, although the bones are heavy, the whole human skeleton is relatively very light. Thus, the weight of a complete woman's skeleton of 5 feet 3 inches is between 11 to 13 pounds. We can never plead a heavy bone structure as an excuse for being overweight.

THE WELL-SHAPED MAN

The chest should be the widest and the thickest part of the body. The muscles of the limbs should be well visible. The shoulders should stand out well away from the chest, and should be well curved.

The lower jaw should join the neck at a definite angle, with no double chin.

There are three signs which indicate that there is no undue growth of fat:

- There should be a muscular projection where the trunk joins the hip-bone: that of the large oblique abdominal muscle, which you never see in a sedentary person.
- The stomach should remind one of the shape of a violin, rounded below by the folds of the

groin. The projections of the two large muscles of the abdomen would correspond to the sound-holes of the violin.

- The two grooves, back and front, running from the fork of the breastbone to the navel and from the shoulders to the loins, should be visible and not thickened by fat.

THE WELL-SHAPED WOMAN

Let us turn now to the ideal shape for a woman. She should be more rounded and softer than a man. In a woman, the sub-cutaneous fat is usually thicker, and the muscles and the bones are less prominent. The connective tissue, and not the muscles, mould a woman's figure. Her body is less bulky and more slender than a man's. Her chest is narrower, thinner and less muscular.

While her waist is narrower, her loins and hips are fuller. In women, the trunk is like a vase standing on the wider pedestal of the hips. But in man the vase appears to overlap the pedestal slightly. Her limbs are not so bulky and do not have muscular contours. Her shoulders are neater and more sloping. The bony projection of her shoulder is more marked.

Her pelvis is lower than a man's. It looks wider because of the relative narrowness of her waist and the lesser development of her thighs.

Although a degree of plumpness is normally present, this should not be at the expense of the bony projections and the principle muscles. Her collar-bones should stand out slightly; the small dips (the collar-bone hollows) above them, of which they mark the lower boundary, are no more a sign of thinness than the fact that the ridge of her tibia shows through the skin of the leg. It's a sign of overweight if you can no longer see the collar-bones.

Her stomach should be flat. Her hips-bone should show through the skin, as should the edges of the lowest ribs. This is not so in the case of her hip joints and the lowest vertebrae, which should be slightly "cushioned."

In the lower limbs, we should guess, rather than actually see, the main muscular lines. Her calves should not show the overdeveloped muscles so common in dancers. They should be slim and not bulgy. Her ankles must be neat, blending gently into the lower part of the calf. The joints of her lower limbs, both knees and ankles, should be slim.

While the thighs should be completely together when you stand bolt upright (nothing is more unsightly than the triangle of light which appears at the top of the thighs between the legs in thin people), this should not be because their inside surfaces are padded with fat, which frequently happens with cellulitics.

The neck should have a clean line and never be scraggy. There should normally be a groove at the nape running up to the back of the head. Where there is undue fattening, this groove fills up with layers of fat, most prominent at the base of the neck.

The face should be well filled-out. The breasts should be sufficiently fat to be rounded although not too large or they may droop. The same applies to the buttocks.

The ideal shape which I have just described is the right of every young woman. It can and should also be that of the older woman, even of the mother of many children whom she has breast-fed, if she knows how to take the necessary precautions.

NORMAL VARIATIONS IN WEIGHT

It is normal for weight to vary in different individuals. We must appreciate this fact if we are to assess the results of cures at their true value.

The daily rhythm

Everyone's weight varies in the course of the day, depending on what he takes in, what he gets rid of and what he uses up on exercise. All this seems obvious enough. These factors however, have an unpredictable influence and, in any case, do not explain by themselves variations in weight.

Our weight is at its lowest when we wake up in

the morning. It is often more than a whole pound lower than it was the night before. This difference can be only partly explained by night losses.

Meals increase weight, but only temporarily, for, by the very fact that they give rise to increased nutritional exchanges, they bring about a sudden fall in weight. This fall partly compensates for the additional weight of the meal. If we don't eat enough this stimulation of nutritional exchanges, ending up in an actual loss of weight, reduces its activity in order to economize the body's resources. This is what happens with animals that hibernate. So, thanks to the compensatory orders given by our junction, providing it is working properly, the increase in our weight is by no means proportionate to the weight of our food intake.

I often quote an amusing experience to my patients. I invited some half-a-dozen friends to a test meal. Each was weighed before the meal, holding a tray carrying the whole of his meal both solid and liquid. The conversation was animated and the arguments heated. Then I re-weighed each of them after the meal, again holding the tray, but this time with nothing but its pattern on it.

There could be no doubt: what was no longer outside had gone inside. Everyone ought to have weighed almost the same to an ounce, as barely an hour had elapsed between the two weighings.

None of my guest was *the same weight as he had been beforehand!* Some had gained an ounce or two, others had lost them. Was this the result of food intake (or the arguments), oxidization, perspiration, or (the opposite) taking in the humidity of the atmosphere? A mystery!

Now let us tackle the question of exercise. True, it slims you, but only under certain conditions.

Two things make you slim, that is to say, cause dissimilation to prevail over assimilation. They are: complete rest for watery overweight, and intense sweaty exercise for fatty overweight. Moderate physical exercise is effective against cellulitis.

From all this we can draw three short conclusions:

- Meals and excretions have less effect on daily weight than in generally supposed.
- Weight usually increases towards the evening (for really "fat" people rather less if they indulge in intense exercise which makes them perspire).
- The night's rest largely supplements the part played by nightly losses in causing one's weight to be at its minimum in the morning.

These factors (meals, excretions and exercises) are not entirely the only factors at work. There are the effects of emotion, irritation and nervous fatigue.

These bring about losses or gains in weight which are often as spectacular as they are inexplicable.

This is the cycle of a middle-aged, balanced individual. In extreme youth, assimilation clearly exceeds excretion. A baby gains an ounce a day. In old age, excretion prevails: the result, a loss of weight.

The weekly rhythm

Excessive week-end activity may be grafted on to the daily rhythm. There are sportsmen who wear themselves out on days when they ought to be resting. And then there are big family meals on Sundays with their procession of digestive upsets.

The monthly rhythm

Women have normal fluctuations in weight especially during the time of their periods. I prefer them to weigh themselves only once a month, on a definite day. Their weight begins to increase in the 3 days immediately before the onset of their period, being a pound or so more when their period starts. At this same time they often feel thirsty. This weight is kept up, because of less urination during the period, then falls and returns to its usual level within four days after the end of the menstrual flow.

When this return to the normal level does not occur (as happens in cases of watery overweight), the woman gains several ounces every period, and thus becomes progressively fatter.

Along with the weight, the hip, midriff and waist measurements increase by half-an-inch to an inch as the period approaches. This corrects itself after the period is over. These increases, which are disproportionate to the woman's usual weight, result from additional water being carried in the subcutaneous tissues at the time of the period.

OVERWEIGHT

A fat surplus of 8% to 15%, over the normal weight, must be considered as *overweight*. Beyond that it is *obesity*. Over 30%, extreme obesity.

Overweight, does not necessarily involve any disorganization of or harm to the system.

Well, you may say, anyone can see when they are getting fat. That's not quite true. Some women delight in being what they call "plump" when they are already truly overweight. *It does also happen the other way round. There are many women who want to slim when there is no reason to do so.*

OBESITY

There is no need to describe the distinguishing marks of obesity. Alas, they are all too obvious. Those unhappy creatures who suffer from it need no description of its discomforts and unsightliness to enable them to recognize it.

The "little plump woman," happy in her plumpness, has only to look in almost any shop or street at the really corpulent members of her sex to realize the risk she is running and yet she sees only the outside. She cannot tell the harm done to the bodily organs or the unhappiness resulting from this condition.

THE WARNING SIGNALS

Overweight begins as "good living". The face grows round and rosy. Everyone agrees that the candidate for obesity is "in fine shape". He is a good match for his wife who may well have the same table habits and be travelling along the same road. Her skirt-belt may be getting a little tight, and perhaps there is a bit of a strain on his jacket-buttons, but this stage is still one of optimism and flourishing health. And at this point no one worries and not even one glance is cast at this book in the bookshop window. Still less likely are they to go off and consult their doctor, but they are making a mistake because things will continue to develop relentlessly. They will get a tummy and a paunch, and larger brassieres will be needed. Shoulders will get plump and the hollows over the collar-bones will disappear completely. This is nothing to be pleased about. No pretty woman should entirely lose these hollows.

Fat will overhang the hips and the waist will disappear. The buttocks will enlarge. The girdle will squeeze the flesh, rolls of which will swell out above and below it. The neck will thicken and lose its normal contour. Just a bit more weight, and appears the double chin. The roll of fat under the nape of the neck will follow.

The skin loses its firm and taut yet supple appearance. It gets puffy and it quivers.

Without wishing, as we said, to elaborate on this picture and come to a sorry sight of breasts sagging down to the stomach, of the stomach drooping over the pubis, of the pubis swelling modestly over the genital organs—let me merely point out that for anyone who is not on the look-out, over weight marches on relentlessly towards obesity.

Be on your guard! There are still pauses in the march towards obesity, even if you don't change your diet. These respites are dangerous tricksters, for they lull the future victim into a false sense of security.

Chapter IV

Beware of Illness

We cannot insist on this too much: overweight not only affects your looks, but your **health** too.

While established obesity actually damages the health, overweight usually causes only discomfort. It is not going outside our scope to stress strongly that obesity, from the strictly medical point of view, is a source of serious dangers, and we must mention them.

Circulation troubles are the most important and serious of these. The obese person gets palpitations, experiences pains in the heart, and becomes extremely out of breath on making the least effort. All these symptoms are not purely due to the body weight that has to be carried about, although this is also an important factor when you realize that every effort made during the day is handicapped by a load of may be twenty to fifty pounds.

Moreover, the heart itself gets tired, because it is burdened by the fat surrounding it, and because the very substance of the heart muscle is impregnated with this fat. Such a heart is at the mercy of the smallest failure.

In the majority of cases, these heart troubles will be associated with arteriosclerosis and high blood pressure, possibly with diabetes or gout. When the weight problem is dealt with and the patients slim down, because they have become aware of the serious nature of their affliction, these troubles will disappear. Otherwise they will take hold, bringing in their train a whole range of potential dangers, apoplexy, paralysis, coronarythrombosis, uraemia due to kidney failure.

As for those of you who are not obese but merely nicely rounded and who look upon yourselves as free from these dangers, you must know that you are a heart-case in the making. Does not any effort, any emotion, make you flush, make your eyes bulge, make you breathless? If this is the case then watch out. Big troubles are lying in wait! Get treatment at once—and get effective treatment. It is no longer a matter of beauty but of health.

Psychological and nervous troubles are common afflictions amongst obese people. The congestive obese types, with red faces, are usually irritable and impulsive. They are energetic in their work, at any rate at first. Whereas the pale ones tend to be apathetic and lethargic, and they tire quickly. We shall see later that most congestive obese people are fatty overweights and the pale obese people are more likely to be watery overweights. Obese people are subject to nervous instability. We find a large proportion of the melancholics, the unstable and the worriers belong to this type.

Does this mean that if you have a continual and irrational fear of impending misfortune you must swallow all sorts of sedatives? Not at all. Get rid of your surplus fat and you will probably regain your calm and balance.

Digestive troubles are usually the result of the intemperance of the obese, rather than of their weight.

Dilation of the stomach, painful digestion, inflammation and spasms of the intestines and congestion of the liver can be accounted for in this way. It is only in the very advanced stage when the fat invades the actual substance of the liver, and causes fatty degeneration like that of the liver of forcibly-fed geese, that it causes digestive upsets in itself.

Be reminded of a serious complaint that can threaten the obese: *diabetes*, which will sometimes disappear completely as soon as sensible dieting brings the weight back to normal.

Genital disorders are rarely absent. Although heart trouble is the most serious, we can say the genital disorders are the dominating factor in the mind of the sufferer, particularly where men are concerned.

The infiltration of fat into the nervous and glandular tissues which control sexual appetite can cause impotence. This may be only temporary, but if it is left too long the cells may mortify. When slimming, taken in time frees these cells from the clutches of fat, they will regain their vitality and sexual desire will return.

For both men and women, sexual troubles disappear under treatment and the glands regain their vitality. This is especially so in the case of the woman who thinks she is sterile but after slimming finds she is pregnant. The low intensity of the menstrual flow (or even its disappearance) could have caused her to make this mistake.

Chapter V

Fatty Overweight

This is found particularly in men. The increase in weight is spread uniformly over the whole body. An extreme example of it is the enormous size of Japanese wrestlers. It is often more noticeable over the upper half of the body (head, neck, arms and trunk) than on the lower limbs. There is both an excess of fat and overdevelopment of muscles. This is not really solely fatty overweight. It could be called "energetic overweight". A type of over worked chemical factory. Enormous stocks are being taken in, consumed and replaced at a giddy speed. Such men are good eaters and this type of overweight could also be termed "feeding overweight". The speed of consumption although fast, cannot cope with the very large food supplies. It is a question of over-activity, not in the sense of physical exercise but of internal reactions—in a word metabolism.

At the outset, the junction tries to deal with the flood of food by speeding up organic consumption, but if the large intake continuous a "bottleneck" in the metabolism is eventually created, with the result that too great quantities have to be put into reserve.

This overweight has its dangers. It is true that such people are usually pleasing to look at. The "fat man" who feels well generally lives well. He is a gourmet and he loves wine. He is jovial, gay, with ruddy face. His eyes light up at the sight of an old Burgundy or a creamed chicken. He is a fine guest, a jolly good fellow who loves life and its pleasures. He is even energetic, though his weight makes him breathless. He is a lady's man, or at any rate he talks a lot about women. But let's turn to the other side of the coin. This is far less attractive—he likes them less than he pretends, his capacity is reduced, his sexual appetite is falling off.

It is just this over-active man who is likely to be the victim of serious complications, precisely because of his internal and external over-activity. He spends his energy extravagantly, in the worst sense of the word: he consumes like a furnace and burns the candle at both ends. Is it his fault? Or rather, is it still his fault? Perhaps not. He is caught in a vicious circle from which he cannot escape. He has a large body to feed, and his mouth is like the mouth of a furnace, always waiting for another shovelful of coal. Hence the dangers which threaten him—arteriosclerosis, the price to be paid for this factory's big turnover, cholesterol, gout, stones, hypertension, coronary thrombosis, diabetes.

SOME CAUSES

The part played by heredity. Often there is a family tendency to stoutness. Professor Marcel Labbe has however taken the view that this is more often the inheritance of the habit of overeating rather than a truly genetic factor.

The part played by age. Some people who have been able to eat excessively with impunity up to a certain age, find that when they reach maturity, they become dangerously obese. This may be caused by poorer functioning of the system and the weaker defence reaction: the result is ageing.

The part played by over-eating. Here we come to the *main factor*. It cannot be denied that excess weight in relation to size is the result of taking in too many calories with food and consequently building up a reserve in the form of an overdeveloped layer of fat.

As this overfeeding is usually due to inability to control a large appetite, you can imagine how useful it would be to be able to control this appetite artificially.

The part played by a sedentary life. This is the logical complement of over-eating. If we store up fattening substances, it is not only because we are absorbing too much but also because we are using up relatively too little by not taking enough muscular exercise. I would add that being sedentary can cause constipation, which is not an insignificant factor in overweight.

The part played by nervous factors. (See nervous overweight, p. 5)

The part played by your glands. Note that when *fatty* overweight is accompanied by a glandular symptoms (difficult periods, etc.) in the great majority of cases the latter are *the effects and not the cause:* they usually disappear when obesity is cured.

In this type of overweight, however, over-secretion by part of the subrenal glands is thought to play a major role.

THE TREATMENT OF FATTY OVERWEIGHT

Above all, reduce your intake of food thereby reducing the amount of fat put in reserve. Although the retention of water is not as important here as in water obesity, it is nonetheless significant, and here too one must combat it to some extent.

Dieting

This is the essential part of the treatment. What is needed is a *quantity* diet on the one hand (that is an overall reduction of the amount of food) and a *quality* diet on the other (affecting mainly the fat producing foods).

The first thing to do is to lower the number of calories taken daily to about 1300 to 1600 calories every 24 hours. See the table of calories value. Cut out fat and alcohol. Reduce carbohydrates to a minimum, but retain a sufficient amount of protein for your own needs (1 oz. per 60 lb. body weight).

Theoretically your meals should be weighed. You should have the following for breakfast, according to their calorie rating:

- 1/4 oz. protein,
- 1/6 oz. fat,
- and 3/4 oz. carbohydrates

On the same principle, each of the two main meals should include:

- 1 oz. protein,
- 3/8 oz. fat
- $1^3/_4$ oz. carbohydrates.

To follow this method, always have by you either at table giving the calorific values of foods, or a table giving their composition in basic products.

We are under no illusion about the difficulty of making such calculations and detailed thinking, and believe it better to give a list of permitted and forbidden foods. Make a point of having regular and balanced meals and obviously you must arrange the following menus according to what is in season.

First assault diet (15 days)

To lose from 8 lb. to 10 lb.

- **Breakfast:** unsugared tea and skimmed milk, 1 or 2 unpeeled apples or a little stewed fruit or yoghurt.
- **11.30:** a large glass of diuretic water.
- **Lunch:** a large bowl of green salad seasoned with vinegar, pepper and liquid paraffin. Either: 5 oz. of grilled meat (unsalted), boiled fish, ham or 2 eggs, then 6 oz. of unsalted boiled vegetables (non-starchy) 1 or 2 apples or other fruit.
- **6 p.m.:** a large glass of diuretic water or skimmed milk.
- **Dinner:** a dish of raw vegetables (same seasoning) 8 oz. green vegetables and fruit.
- **Before going to bed:** a large glass of skimmed milk.

  N.B. — You can interchange lunch and dinner but take no bread, biscuits, cake, salt or sugar, and do not drink during meals. *Never miss a meal.*

On the 8th and 15th days of the first assault diet, try a day on a milk diet, spending the day in bed or in a comfortable armchair if possible:

- **8 a.m.:** 1/2 pint diluted skimmed milk and 2 grated unpeeled apples.
- **10 a.m.:** 1/4 pint diuretic water.
- **1 p.m.:** 3/4 pint skimmed milk, with 2 grated apples.
- **5 p.m.:** 1/2 pint diuretic water.
- **8 p.m.:** 3/4 pint skimmed milk, with 2 grated apples.

Follow-up diet (2 months)

To lose: 10 lb. a month in weight

- Breakfast will consist entirely of a little tea or coffee with a dash of milk and 1 or 2 apples or half a grapefruit.
- It is absolutely forbidden to drink while eating. Eat very little salted food.
- Cut out completely bread, biscuits, cake, preserves and sugar.
- Take a large glass of diuretic water on rising, at 11 a.m. and at 6 p.m.
- Have one day of milk diet (see first assault) every 10 days.

MONDAY (1st and 3rd weeks)

- **Lunch:** salad of raw vegetables grated or chopped thin (carrots, lettuce, beans, a few peas, a little cabbage, radish, asparagus tips, olives, tomatoes according to the season), 1 dessertspoonful of wheat germ, 2 fried eggs, 1/2 grapefruit, black coffee.
- **Dinner:** half a lettuce, 2 small cream cheese, 1 orange.

TUESDAY (1st and 3rd)

- **Lunch:** 1/2 grapefruit or melon, 1 spoonful wheat germ, 1 portion lambs kidney, leeks, 1 orange, black coffee.
- **Dinner:** celery, 3 oz. Dutch cheese, stewed apples.

WEDNESDAY (1st and 3rd)

- **Lunch:** salad of raw vegetables, wheat germ, 3 ozs. calves liver, chicory, grapes or pear, black coffee.
- **Dinner:** carrots, 6 oz. of yoghurt, stewed plums or prunes.

THURSDAY (1st and 3rd)

- **Lunch:** 1/2 grapefruit, wheat germ, 2 poached eggs with tomato sauce or 12 oysters, green beans, apple, black coffee.
- **Dinner:** 1 lettuce, cottage cheese, 1 orange.

FRIDAY (1st and 3rd)

- **Lunch:** salad of raw vegetables, wheat germ, sole, aubergine (egg plant), 2 slices of pineapple, black coffee.
- **Dinner:** leeks, 6 oz. yoghurt, 1 apple or grapes.

SATURDAY (1st and 3rd)

- **Lunch:** 1/2 grapefruit, wheat germ, a grilled fillet steak, 1 artichoke, 1 orange, black coffee.
- **Dinner:** chicory, cheese, pear.

SUNDAY (1st and 3rd)

- **Lunch:** salad of raw vegetables, wheat germ, 5 oz. poultry or rabbit, 1 lettuce, 1 small cream cheese, black coffee.
- **Dinner:** green beans, cheese, 2 slices of pineapple.

MONDAY (2nd and 4th weeks)

- **Lunch:** 1/2 grapefruit, wheat germ, crab or lobster, artichoke, 1 orange black coffee.
- **Dinner:** 1 lettuce, 6 oz. yoghurt, stewed apples.

TUESDAY (2nd and 4th)

- **Lunch:** salad of raw vegetables, wheat germ, 1/4 lb. beefsteak, 1/2 grapefruit, 1 apple, black coffee.
- **Dinner:** boiled macaroni or spaghetti without butter, cream cheese, stewed prunes.

WEDNESDAY (2nd and 4th)

- **Lunch:** 1/2 grapefruit, wheat germ, 1 slice roast lamb, cooked tomatoes, 1 orange, black coffee.
- **Dinner:** one small potato, cheddar cheese, egg custard.

THURSDAY (2nd and 4th)

- **Lunch:** salad of raw vegetables, wheat germ, 1/4 lb. veal, 1 lettuce, 1 pear, black coffee.
- **Dinner:** leeks in white sauce; 6 oz. yoghurt, 1 orange.

FRIDAY (2nd and 4th)

- **Lunch:** 1/2 grapefruit, wheat germ, 1 portion of white fish, 1 boiled potato, 2 fresh figs, black coffee.
- **Dinner:** chicory, gruyere cheese, pear or grapes.

SATURDAY (2nd and 4th)

- **Lunch:** salad of raw vegetables, wheat germ, a slice of ham, spinach, stewed prunes, black coffee.
- **Dinner:** celery, 2 oz. cheddar cheese, 1 apple.

SUNDAY (2nd and 4th)

- **Lunch:** 1/2 grapefruit, wheat germ, 1 portion of chicken, asparagus, 2 slices of pineapple, black coffee.

- **Dinner:** carrots, gruyere cheese, 1 orange.

After the the two months on the follow-up diet, have one day one the skimmed milk diet and then go on to three months of the consolidation diet.

Consolidation diet (3 months)

No more reducing. Just consolidate your achievement. No more restrictions as to quantity; but do be sensible, that's all.

The food you may eat

Non-fatty soups, vegetable broths, without bread and only slightly salted.

Beef, veal and mutton, taken from the lean part of the animal.

Lean fish: cod, trout, sole, plaice etc. without sauce or butter,

Shell fish.

Lean poultry.

Ham.

Eggs (1 a day, maximum).

Fresh butter and liquid paraffin in small quantities.

Fresh or condensed milk, skimmed and unsweetened.

Fresh cheeses, with low fat content.

Macaroni, spaghetti or potatoes in very small quantities.

All green vegetables cooked or raw.

All fruits, raw or stewed, without sugar.

Salt in very small quantity.

Fruit juices, herbal teas, light wines, preferably white.

You must **never drink while eating.** The only exception: one glass of wine once a week at the most.

The food you may not eat

Above all and absolutely forbidden: **bread and biscuits, pastries and jam** (no exceptions allowed).

Fatty soups.

Fat meats, fat poultry (goose, etc.)

Fatty fish (mackerel, herrings, turbot, salmon).

Meat in sauces and stews.

High game.

Fat pork meats (liver sausage, potted meats, black-pudding, sausages, salt pork).

Fried foods.

Offal, liver pate, tinned meat, smoked fish, caviar.

Lard, margarine, butter, oil.

Cream and milk foods.

Cornflakes, starch, flour, semolina, tapioca, rice.

Fatty, fermented and salted cheeses.

Dried vegetables, mushrooms, sauerkraut.

Bananas, chestnuts, walnuts, jam, syrup, honey, cocoa, chocolate.

Wine, beer cider and all kinds of alcoholic or sweetened drinks.

In order to choose from the various foods those which have the lowest calorie content, you can glance from time to time at the table given below.

THE CALORIE VALUE OF FOODS

	Oz.	Calories
Beverages		
Beer, half-pint		100
Wine, one glass		70
Milk, half-pint		200
Tea, without mild		0
Tea, with milk		10
Coffee, without milk		0
Cocoa, half milk		112
Fish		
White fish	1	21
Tinned sardines	1	85
Herring	1	47
Meat		
Bacon	1	128
Beef	1	89

Mutton	1	95
Pork	1	114
Chicken	1	38
Dairy Products		
Butter, or margarine	1	218
Cheese, cheddar	1	120
Egg, standard size	2¼	100
Fruit (medium-size)		
Apple		70
Banana		75
Grapefruit		40
Orange		55
Pear		60
Vegetables		
Beans, runner	2	8
Brussels sprouts	2	20
Cabbage	2	14
Carrot	2	12
Onion	2	12
Lettuce	2	5
Peas	2	34
Potato	2	45
Tomato	2	7

Sundries

Bread, one slice, white or brown or toast	2	144
Biscuits, plain	1	120
Biscuits, sweet	1	126
Cakes, plain	1	89
Flour, white	1	98
Rice	1	102
Sugar	1	108
Jam	1	71

EXERCISES AND GYMNASTICS

Take energetic exercise: physical training, gymnastics exercises and sport of all kinds but if you are really obese you must wait until dieting has slimmed you down.

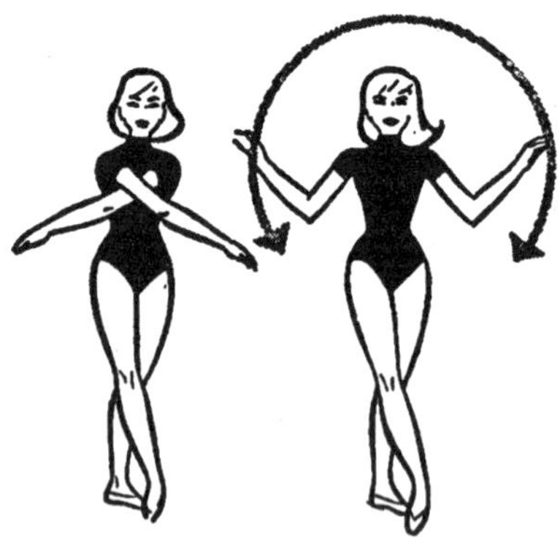

Overweight people must think of their heart and circulation systems which may not stand up to strenuous exercise, and they should consult the doctor first.

See to it that the effect of the exercise is not cancelled out by yielding to the hunger that it causes, and beware of overmuch yielding to the thirst caused by the loss of water by perspiration.

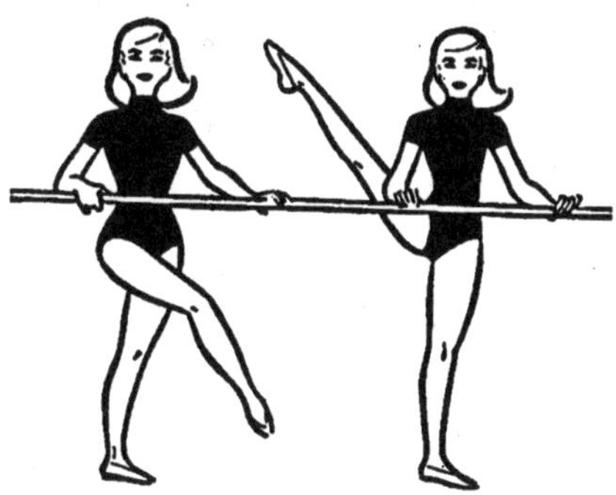

Gentle activities, such as walking, promote assimilation and therefore added weight, and they are *not recommended.*

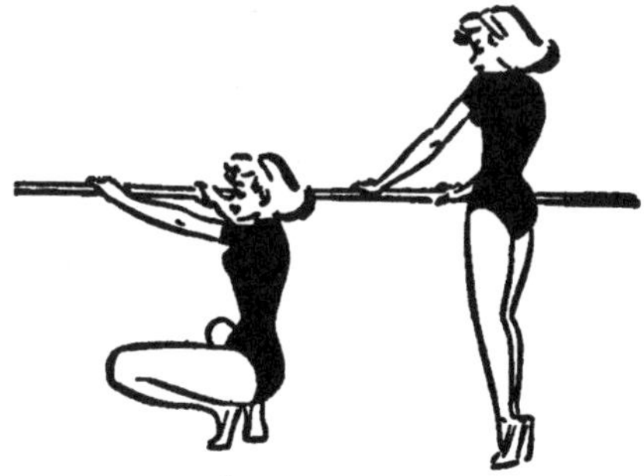

Here are the slimming exercises which Robert Raynaud, a specialist in these matters, has prepared for those afflicted with fatty overweight.

- **Loosening of neck region** by head movements.

A. *Bending forwards and backwards*

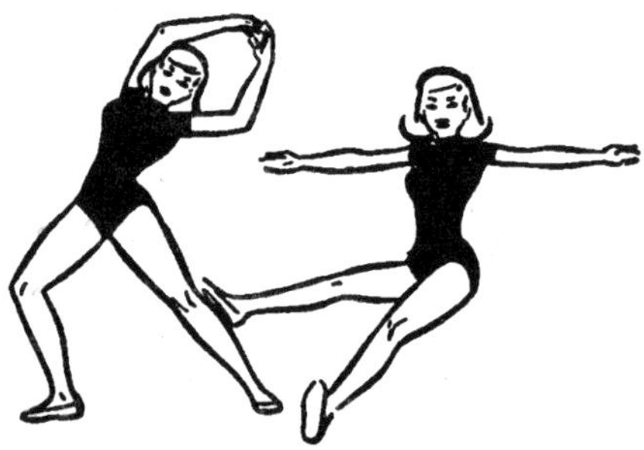

Body upright: lower the head and look at the floor, then raise it and look at the ceiling. *15 to 20 times.*

B. *Twisting*

Turn the head to the left, then to the right, without moving the shoulders. *15 to 20 times.*

C. *Bending sideways.*

Drop the head to the left side, then to the right, without raising the shoulders. *15 to 20 times.*

- **Loosening the shoulders** by circling the arms round in a fairly rapid rhythm.

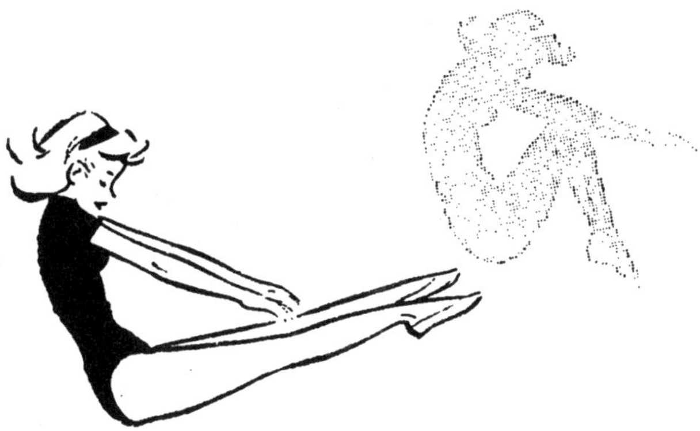

Stand up, arms stretched downwards. Bring the arms together, and cross one over the other. Move the arms upwards in a circular motion, right arm to the left and left arm to the right. Bring them down to the sides and then stretch them backwards as far as you can. *20 to 25 times.*

Loosening the hips. Stand up, grasp a bar or the back of a chair, swing the right leg in front of the left, then kick it up (very loosely) as high as you can towards the right. Do the same with the other leg. *12 to 20 times.*

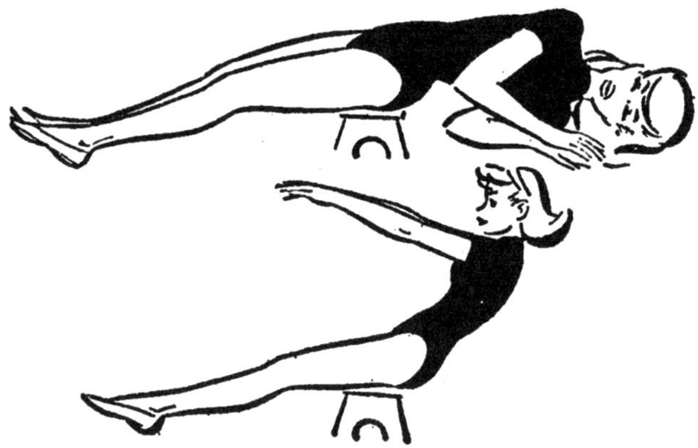

- **Loosening the thighs and knees.** Stand facing a bar or the back of a chair, bend both knees and sit on the heels. Then stand up on tiptoe. *30 to 60 times.*
- **Slimming the ankles.** Stand on tiptoe, lower the heels to the ground and then lift the toes. *40 to 80 times.*
- **Slimming the waist.**

A. Legs stretched apart, fingers clasped above the head. Lower the trunk to the left, bending the right leg; and then to the right, bending your left leg. *10 to 20 times each side.*

B. Sit on the ground, legs stretched apart, trunk upright, arms stretched out to the sides. Swing the trunk to the right, then to the left, keeping the arms stretched in line. *20 to 30 times.*

- **Abdominal toning up.**

A. Sit on the floor, balanced on the buttocks. Bring the trunk forward and bend the knees, then return to the starting position. A rowing movement *20 to 30 times.*

B. Sit on a low stool, with feet wedged under a chair. Bend the trunk backwards and touch the floor with one shoulder, turning the trunk to bring the two shoulders into a vertical plane. Lift the trunk and return to the sitting position. *12 to 15 times, alternating.*

- **Finish by jumping.** Hop twice on the left foot while kicking the right foot forward; then twice on the right foot while kicking the left foot forward. *15 to 20 times.*

TO ELIMINATE EXCESS WATER

Whatever the method, the principle is the same: water is "sucked out" of the cell spaces and in order to re-impregnate the tissue with their normal quota of water, the body must obtain it by destroying fats. All this only happens, of course, if you have drunk nothing in the meantime. If you have, the body takes the water from the digestive tubes and leaves the fats intact and then the whole process has to start again.

There are various ways of "sucking out" a large amount of water in order to eliminate it.

The first, by drugs, consists of *purging*. This causes water to be absorbed into the intestines. The disadvantage of this is, that if repeated often, it irritates the intestinal walls.

The second consists of the use of *diuretics*.

The third is *sudation*, or sweating.

The ordinary sweating process is natural perspiration as a result of exercise (physical training and sports). You must of course take care to see that you do not tire your heart.

Then there is the inducing of sweat by artificial means.

This also can tire the heart, though to a lesser degree, by speeding up its movement. But this danger need not be exaggerated. Only those with heart trouble need to refrain from using these methods.

Since they are very well known and in general use, we need only merely mention foam and paraffin baths Finnish saunas, Turkish baths, slimming garments and such artificial means of making the body sweat away excess water.

These methods are a valuable help to people who want to do more than just diet, but it is quite impossible to slim solely by such measures as these. The loss of a lb. or two which they cause is merely a loss of water, and therefore a temporary dehydration which brings on intense thirst.

If the patient then slakes his thirst, he loses all the benefits of the treatment.

If on the other hand, he is strong-willed enough to resist his thirst the body, in the absence of a simpler solution, will have to seek its water, at least partly, by burning up some of the accumulation of fat.

DRUGS

When you are on a strict diet the discomfort of hunger can be minimised by drugs, but these are not to be used when the patient is not a naturally big eater or if he can control his appetite without too much difficulty. Moreover, they must be absorbed long enough before a meal (at least an hour) to give their anti-hunger action time to develop.

These appetite-reducing "psychamines" are available in pill form. Your doctor will advise you about them. The modern reducers cause far fewer secondary complications (such as insomnia and palpitations) than earlier medicines of the kind.

If you don't feel strong enough to endure dieting by yourself, if you want to "reduce without tears," drugs can help you to put up with the necessary restrictions cheerfully.

These drugs-like many others-may, if taken uninterruptedly, prove habit-forming. You must avoid this by going without them for 10 days each month and relying on your willpower during that time to avoid any excess. Your doctor will take advantage of this pause to increase your urinary output by means of diuretic drugs.

Should you go on taking these drugs for a long time or permanently? Does their effect cease when you stop taking them?

Certainly not. Nevertheless, these drugs have to be taken for several months, even if the patient has recovered normal weight. What the body has to do is to develop new feeding habits, to get used to a certain ration of food. Once this stage is reached, cut out the drugs. The patient will then find it easy to stabilize his or her weight by means of a light diet.

Can anyone take these drugs?

No! Neurotics, heart sufferers and some other people must not take them. Here again, only your doctor can decide.

Moreover, these drugs are usually available only on a doctor's prescription. *It must be emphasised that a doctor's advice whenever drugs enter the picture is vital.*

These drugs can cause damage if not taken correctly, on proper medical advise.

There are some preparations which aim to cut down the appetite mechanically by distending the stomach and thus giving a feeling of fullness.

Useful auxiliary medicines are those which help to correct internal laziness. The easy functioning of the bowels is most important, and a gentle laxative should be used in such cases.

PSYCHOLOGICAL TREATMENT

Emotional shock can be a cause of overweight. This can upset the working of the "junction," occasioning watery overweight by provoking hunger pangs of a paroxysmal and obsessional nature. This must be fought by personal determination, with the help, if necessary, of a specialist. Psychamine drugs can be of great assistance. The slight feeling of exhilaration they cause helps the patient to forget the attractions of the table.

In some obstinate cases, however, it is necessary to resort to psycho-analysis.

HYDRO-THERMAL TREATMENTS

These are recommended as a useful auxiliary means of getting rid of superfluous weight.

You are fat-prone if...

- You like to eat very well-and do!
- You have rather sedentary habits or a sedentary job.
- You put on weight during holidays (if you take things easy).
- Emotional upsets and worry make you lose weight.
- Massage and douches have little effect.
- You are "short-winded" but, apart from this, you are dynamic, very active and are fond of good living.
- Sweating sessions cause moderate but lasting loss of weight.
- Cutting down on your food (especially bread and cakes) has a noticeable effect.
- Overweight has overtaken you at a time other than at a stage of sexual development (puberty, menopause, pregnancy).
- The overweight affects the upper part of your body (arms-shoulders-face) as much as or more than the lower part.
- Overweight is accompanied by circulation trouble.
- You rarely feel cold.

In which case, what should you do about it?

- Weigh yourself every 28 days.
- Cut down on your food, and cut out, in particular, biscuits, bread, cakes. Use little salt and no sugar.
- Breakfast on tea and apples.
- Don't drink while you are eating.
- If necessary, reduce your appetite by taking psychamines and hour before meals.
- If they are available, take foam baths or Turkish baths.
- 20 minutes of physical exercises preceded by muscular limbering up, every morning. Energetic sports.
- Drink diuretic water.
- Consult you doctor.

You must never...

- Weigh yourself very frequently.
- Lose patience.
- Let yourself become constipated.
- Take drugs of your own accord *and without medical supervision.*

Chapter VI

Watery Overweight

Most women we think of as fat are really female sponges. Watery overweight is one of the commonest forms of female overweight. In fact, it is almost exclusively female. Gilbert Dreyfus described it as *spongy obesity.* Albeaux-Fernet as *hydro-lipopexy* and de Gennes as *paradoxical obesity*. It is in fact a unique syndrome characterised by retention of fat and water together, but with the water predominating.

The main characteristic of this type of overweight is that it is paradoxical, in the sense that unlike the ordinary overweight we have earlier described, it cannot be explained by overeating. Sixty-five percent of European women put on weight during the war years when food was rationed.

How to spot watery overweight

This type of excess weight occurs almost solely in women, sometimes in young women, but more often still in the young girl who is just entering the early years of adulthood with all the difficulties these bring. It may also occur at the menopause.

Over a period which may vary from several months to two years, the scales may show an increase of as much as from 15 to 25 lb. or even more. If you ask the young woman how much she eats, you will not be too surprised to learn that far from overeating, she is subjected to the family's gibes about how little she eats. Often she deliberately goes without food and drinks only very little. Some European women who were deported to concentration camps increased in weight in spite of the dreadful privations they experienced?

The odd thing about this type of excess weight is that it affects the upper limbs and the chest relatively little. Rather it predominates over the lower half of the body, the hips and the buttocks. From there, it extends to the stomach, the thighs and the inside of the knees.

Further, the patient complains of cold feet and hands and cannot get them warm in bed. If you look at them, you will see that they are red and damp. Often chilblains occur, even in summer.

Moreover, red blotches appear on the legs which, in addition to their unattractive increase in size, begin to get rough, coarse-grained, veined and stiff. They hurt when they are touched. Then the leg is as cold as the foot and also often has the same painful chilblains. The patient complains of a frequently twisted ankle. The nails break or split.

A vital point, in nearly all cases, the periods are irregular. Although warning of them is given long in advance by intestinal swelling, a painful tension in the chest and nervousness, they are late, are slight, or sometimes are not evident at all. In any event, they are irregular and frequently painful and they last only 2 or 3 days. They are often accompanied by headaches.

These troubles have a serious effect on the general condition. The young girl is exhausted by the least effort and drags herself about, chronically tired. This leads us to one of the outstanding characteristics of watery overweight; namely, that whatever causes repercussions on the nervous system (physical or mental strain, worry, emotional shocks) increases weight and volume, while relaxation and rest diminish it (the favourable influence of holidays).

THE MECHANICS OF WATERY OVERWEIGHT

The exchange of moisture

Do you remember that amusing experiment of the testmeals I described in the chapter on "normal weight-variations". My guests showed seemingly abnormal weight variations in the space of an hour?

Actually, the gains and losses could have occurred in only one way—the passage of water in the form of vapour through the skin in one direction or the other, according to whether there was a loss or a gain. This brought to light a vital fact. Apart from what we normally take in, reject, or sweat out in the form of perspiration, we are perpetually exchanging water with the outside atmosphere. This purely gaseous exchange, though unseen, is tremendous. It can be around 2 pints of **liquid** a day.

Normally, we absorb moisture at certain times of the day and then invisibly reject it at others, but we have found that the successive phases end up by cancelling one another out and balancing every 24 hours. This occurs where the invaporation equals the evaporation. The latter is an invisible perspiration which can be seen only if we cover ourselves with a rubber or plastic garment.

And so every day, for a person who is well balanced from both the nerve and glandular points of view, the assets equal the liabilities. There is no balance outstanding either way and the weight remains stable. We have also found that for some people being particularly "spongy". But in the last analysis the result is the same.

On the other hand, if an emotional condition or

upset or a fit of anger occurs, the disturbed "junction" is going to react on the tissues' thirst for water, with the result that within a few hours, and for no apparent reason, many ounces of water will accumulate in the body, moisture intake exceeding moisture out-flow. We have only to retain 7 ounces in every pound that we absorb each day to put on 12 lb. a month without having either eaten or drunk to excess. The woman (since in eight cases out of ten it is a woman) has become a female sponge!

The causes of this overweight

Food. Here, dieting will be as important a part of the treatment as it was in the previous chapter. However, overeating does not *usually* account for overweight at all.

The important factor here, as far as eating is concerned, lies in most cases in the preponderance of a *diet which is rich in water and poor in meat.* Meat does not automatically increase weight. Carnivorous animals are thin. If you question patient, you will find that the diet they usually impose on themselves consists mainly of vegetables, soups and fruits, cutting out meat whose acidifying properties, in small quantities, are necessary for our chemical reactions. This lack of balance in feeding-with "too much water, not enough albumin"-leads to stopping the normal chemical reactions through its alkalising character, and seems to prevent our body getting rid of the surplus water, which then accumulates in the tissues. If you drink a pint of water, you eliminate it altogether. If you drink two pints and are suffering from this kind of complaint, you get rid of no more and you store the remainder. But here again, as with fatty overweight, all patients on the same diet don't react the same way. If all women were to take the same amount of water and meat they would not all retain the same amount of water.

So we are forced to acknowledge that it is the derangement (nervous for instance) or straining (due to a diet too long out of balance) of the delicate and most complex mechanism of the junction which must explain these differences.

Salt also plays a significant part. Salt holds water. Further, at the beginning of menstruation the blood becomes loaded with salt, which explains the retention of water usual at this time. In order to combat, at once and at the same time, the retention of water and thirst, we must strictly limit the intake of salt.

Exercise plays as important a part here as in the previous chapter, but the *other way around.* It is absolutely contraindicated here, as is walking or gymnastics. It causes you to put on weight, whereas rest and lying down reduce weight considerably.

Age is also very important. Paradoxical overweight occurs especially at times of sexual development and change. A young woman can expect an improvement with marriage, and again with her first pregnancy, apart from the treatments we are going to recommend. At the menopause, a woman can expect her circulatory condition to become stable.

Endocrine factors. It is in fact a matter of phases of sexual development rather than age. The theory that the retention of water in the tissues, owing to a decrease in urinary elimination, is encouraged, not only by lack of balance in food intake, but also by ovarian or pituitary activity, seems to have many other arguments in its favour, namely:

- This type of obesity concerns women almost exclusively.
- Normal women usually gain a little weight, about a lb. when their period starts, and lose that when it is over. In cases of watery overweight, this loss does not occur. So the woman puts on weight successively at each monthly period.
- Œstrogenic hormones increase this overweight in women, and induce abnormal retention of water when used in experiments on guinea-pigs.

- Watery overweight often occurs at a stage of sexual development-puberty, pregnancy, miscarriage, a natural or induced menopause.

Psychological factors. The emotional element will still be in the foreground in these cases. We have mentioned people in concentration camps who put on weight despite their diet. It is obviously in these overweights that the word "paradoxical" has its most dramatic meaning. This is also true of false obesity where we can often see the effect of a severe mental shock.

There is no doubt that worries and strong emotions do sometimes cause what writers have been tempted to denominate as "psychosomatic overweight".

The electro-chemical balance of the body fluids. One final factor seems to act upon this abnormal thirst for water of the subcutaneous and deep connective tissues. It is the electro-chemical balance of the blood and of the resulting lymphatic fluids.

There is evidence, in cases of watery overweight, of a deficiency in the blood of some metallic catalytic agents (zinc, copper, nickel, manganese, or perhaps cobalt) varying from one patient to another.

Treatment by giving very small doses of these metals results in favourable changes in the electrical charges of the different elements in the blood, thereby preventing certain abnormal chemical activities. Of these, the one that concerns us is the sponginess of the tissues.

THE TREATMENT OF WATERY OVERWEIGHT

Diet

We have seen how important unbalanced eating is in the origin of this kind of overweight. The obvious deduction is that dieting must be the leading factor in its treatment.

I shall set out the diet to be followed in its most drastic form, the less established the complaint, the less strict it need be.

But the diet will follow these general principles:

- Never drink with your meals and drink very little between meals.
- Don't salt your food.
- Few vegetables and plenty of meat.
- No watery foods (soup, juicy fruits, melon, etc.)

This, then is *dehydration* diet.

There is also a good case for getting medical advice before embarking on strict diets. Bear this in mind especially with this diet.

Assault treatment (2 months)

This is a very effective diet for severe cases:

It consists, *for 4 consecutive days in each week of:*

1. Eating only protein,
2. Strictly avoiding water and salt.

On the other 3 days, the patient must follow the relative *dehydration* diet set out later.

On these days, drink about a pint of diuretic water a day, part of this to be taken in the morning before eating in order to bring about urinary elimination.

In practice, during the four days of *dry diet,* each of the 3 meals will consist solely of:

- 1 hard-boiled egg or 4 oz. meat,
- 3 oz. cheese,
- two unsalted rusks.

No liquid either during or between meals. No salt.

Remember never follow this diet without consulting your doctor.

During the 4 days of this diet, the patient will lose 6 to 8 lb., but will regain all but a lb. or so during the 3 days of "normal overweight" diet of the rest of the week. Thus there will be a new and permanent loss averaging about a lb. each week, until the weight is back to normal.

This diet must be strictly followed for at least 2 months. This length of time is necessary for creating new habits for the tissues and organs regarding the retention of water. Then, and only then, can this diet be dropped finally without the weight going up again. The improvement then becomes permanent and the false obesity is conquered.

The most curious thing is that this treatment has in it the excellent quality of making the periods regular again, increasing their amount and even starting them again if they have stopped.

We would stress that no additional glandular treatment is necessary to bring about this improvement in the menstrual flow. The dry diet suffices. This proves that lack of balance at the centre is of greater consequence than glandular disorders which, though spectacular, are quite secondary.

There is some risk in this waterless and saltless diet if the kidneys are not absolutely sound. Your kidneys must therefore be carefully watched if you follow it.

If you find it difficult to put up with and, in any case, at the end of 2 months, pass on to the following diet:

The relative dehydration diet (4 months)

Breakfast consists solely of a boiled egg, or of a piece of non-fermented cheese, or yoghurt, or an apple, without bread, and half a cup of black coffee with half a lump of sugar. Cut out bread, biscuits, cakes, jam, preserves and juicy fruits. Don't drink with your meals. Eat very little salted food.

Drink two-thirds of a glass of diuretic water when you get up, at the end of the morning and again at the end of the afternoon. This is the only drink allowed.

Raw vegetable salads may be seasoned with vinegar, liquid paraffin, pepper and diet salt.

MONDAY (1st and 3rd weeks)

- **Lunch:** salad of raw vegetables, 1 slice of ham, 1 small cream cheese, 1 apple, a small cup of tea.
- **Dinner:** 1 lettuce heart, 1 portion of fresh fish (plaice, sole, cod, haddock), 1 yoghurt.

TUESDAY (1st and 3rd)

- **Lunch:** salad of raw vegetables, 1 escalope of veal, Dutch cheese, pineapple, small cup of tea.
- **Dinner:** 1 artichoke, whiting, 1 small cream cheese.

WEDNESDAY (1st and 3rd)

- **Lunch:** salad of raw vegetables, 1 slice of roast lamb, 2 yoghurts (5 to 6 oz.), dried figs, tea.
- **Dinner:** carrots, fresh fish or shell fish, cottage cheese.

THURSDAY (1st and 3rd)

- **Lunch:** salad of raw vegetables, 1 grilled steak, cottage cheese, prunes, tea.
- **Dinner:** 1 lettuce, ham, 1 yoghurt.

FRIDAY (1st and 3rd)

- **Lunch:** salad of raw vegetables, 1 fish steak, 2 yoghurts, stewed apples, tea.
- **Dinner:** pears, grilled fresh herring, 1 cream cheese.

SATURDAY (1st and 3rd)

- **Lunch:** salad of raw vegetables, 2 fried eggs, low fat-content cheese, grapes, tea.
- **Dinner:** tomato juice, cold ham or beef, cream cheese.

SUNDAY (1st and 3rd)

- **Lunch:** salad of raw vegetables, portion of chicken, cottage cheese, pineapple, tea.

- **Dinner:** grilled fish with green beans, Swiss cheese.

MONDAY (2nd and 4th weeks)

- **Lunch:** salad of raw vegetables, 2 hard-boiled eggs with tomato sauce, 2 yoghurts, 1 apple, tea.
- **Dinner:** macaroni or spaghetti cooked in water, 1 fillet of sole, 1 yoghurt.

TUESDAY (2nd and 4th)

- **Lunch:** salad of raw vegetables, 3 oz. calves liver, cream cheese, pineapple, tea.
- **Dinner:** asparagus, 1 fried egg, 1 yoghurt.

WEDNESDAY (2nd and 4th)

- **Lunch:** salad of raw vegetables, lamb's kidneys, Dutch cheese, dried figs, tea.
- **Dinner:** 1 potato, fresh fish, cottage cheese.

THURSDAY (2nd and 4th)

- **Lunch:** salad of raw vegetables, 1/4 lb. grilled steak, Swiss cheese, prunes, tea.
- **Dinner:** 1 lettuce, cold meat, 1 yoghurt.

FRIDAY (2nd and 4th)

- **Lunch:** salad of raw vegetables, 4 oz. fish, Swiss cheese, stewed fruit, tea.

- **Dinner:** spinach, 1 poached egg, 1 small cream cheese.

SATURDAY (2nd and 4th)

- **Lunch:** salad of raw vegetables, 2 boiled eggs, low fat content cheese, grapes, tea.
- **Dinner:** carrots, ham, 1 yoghurt.

SUNDAY (2nd and 4th)

- **Lunch:** salad of raw vegetables, chicken or lobster, Swish cheese, pineapple, tea.
- **Dinner:** salad, cold meat, cottage cheese.

REST

In these cases, exercise, overwork, walking fatigue and late nights encourage overweight. You must relax and rest. Good results are achieved in the most serious cases, simply from *resting in bed.*

This is because a lying-down position causes an increase in urination. This simple mechanism is often enough by itself to cure some patients. Cases are known of young women regularly losing 15 to 20 lb. a week during three weeks in bed.

Science has proved that when these patients are living an "upright" life, not in bed, they pass less water than they drink. But when they spends their time in bed they pass more water, by urination, than they drink. I cannot too strongly advice patients who are going to take this treatment (3 weeks' rest in bed) to combine it with a strict diet so as to make absolutely sure of achieving results. Actually, rest in bed means that the minimum amount of food is being used up, and the patient who doesn't cut down on food will gain in fat what has been lost in water.

GENERAL MASSAGE

Expert massage acts indirectly, by *its effect on the nervous system* (reflex therapeutic massage) and by the relaxation it brings.

HOW TO GET RID OF WATER!

Sweating, laxatives, diuretics

Paradoxically, these are ineffective in cases of *watery* overweight, for which they would seem the obvious and logical answer.

This is easily explained. They cannot bring about a permanent loss of weight in cases of pure watery overweight, as there is no surplus fat to break down. The tissues which are greedy for water and temporarily dehydrated, will merely wait for the first liquid food to "fill up." This is why sweating, laxatives and diuretics are no use.

Water which is artificially removed from tissues that are greedy for it always returns, and quickly. If the body doesn't get fluid, it finds water in the air we breathe.

The only solution is gradually to reduce this abnormal need of the tissues for water:

- By cutting down water intake over a long period and by diminishing the intake of salt,
- By acting on the electro-chemical balance of the blood,
- By acting, as far as possible, on the "junction" (see page 5).

YOU HAVE WATERY OVERWEIGHT IF ....

- You eat moderately. Putting yourself on a vegetable and fruit diet and even cutting down your food considerably makes no difference.
- You are overstraining yourself physically and mentally.
- Rest and relaxation are immediately beneficial.
- Emotion and worry cause you to put on weight.
- You don't feel really well.
- Sweating sessions cause considerable but only temporary losses of weight.
- You have serious trouble with your periods, which diminish or disappear altogether.

- The overweight occurs at the time of a change in sexual development.
- The overweight is predominantly in the lower part of the body, on hips, buttocks and thighs.
- It is accompanied by serious circulation troubles (the legs are veined, dry and rough), the ankles are heavy and swollen by the evening.
- You have chilblains every winter.
- Your nails split, you twist your ankle for no apparent reason.

What can you do?

- Weight yourself every 28 days.
- Cut out bread and cakes, avoid vegetables, juicy fruits, soups. Eat eggs, meat and cheese (unsalted).
- For breakfast eat an egg. Swiss cheese or yoghurt.
- Don't eat and drink at the same time. Drink very little between meals.
- If necessary go on an eggs-meat-cheese diet for 3 to 4 days a week.
- Rest and relax as much as possible.
- Drink mineral waters which encourage total elimination.

What you must not do

- Weigh yourself constantly.
- Lose patience.
- Go without food, or cut out meat and put yourself on vegetables and fruit exclusively.
- Indulge in physical exercise and exhausting sport.
- Go to bed late.
- Take strong purgatives.
- Let yourself get constipated.
- Take drugs without medical supervision.
- Follow a dry diet, which is difficult and sometimes dangerous, without medical supervision.

Chapter VII

Cellulitis

The essential difference between cellulitis and fatty obesity or watery obesity is that it *affects certain limited areas only,* whereas fat and water invade large areas of the body.

Some authors have considered cellulitis to be simply a localized form of watery obesity. They group the two ailments together and so recognize only two main categories.

But cellulitis, even though it is often met with in conjunction with watery overweight, merits separate consideration.

- Because it can, even though rarely, be dissociated from it.
- Because cellulitis has a characteristic of its own, differing from watery overweight and fatty overweight. In both the latter, the skin stretches easily and painlessly.
- Because it has causes peculiar to itself.
- Because its treatment is different.

If we do find it often associated with watery overweight, this is only because its causes often co-exist with the causes of the latter.

A woman with cellulitis may have it only on the hips, or the nape of her neck, or in both legs, the rest of the body being unaffected.

When cellulitis is present at the same time as either of the two generalized forms of obesity, the cellulitis should receive separate and primary treatment.

WHAT IS CELLULITIS?

Cellulitis is an inflammation of the connective tissue caused by poisons accumulating there instead of being thrown out by the body. The most common of these poisons are uric, lastic and oxalic acids.

In cases of cellulitis, the double chin, thick shoulders and swollen ankles are stuffed with organic waste matter which is normally rejected through urine, sweat and bowels. Here "normally" means if you are in good health and are living a healthy life. This waste matter collects in the connective tissue.

THE CONNECTIVE TISSUE

Connective tissue is to be found in the body wherever there are no organs. Under the skin, it is known as subcutaneous cellular tissue, but it is found elsewhere as "filler tissue". It is the binding tissue of the body. Through the agency of the lymphatic vessels it brings food to the organs and carries away the remains of what they have used or consumed.

Inflammation of the connective tissue

In cases of cellulitis, this connective tissue fills with a lymph, containing much waste matter which irritates it and causes it to contract. It then fills with water which the body is prompt to supply in order to dilute the poisoned lymph and relieve the irritation of the tissues. If the process continues, the water thickens into mucus which in turn becomes semi-solid matter. This congests the cellular tissue, which then becomes painful. This is cellulitis.

Eventually there will develop sclerosis or atrophy which is the final stage in the evolution of all inflammatory conditions.

The contraction, which is the initial reaction of the connective tissue, is at the same time the cause of all these misfortunes. The irritation causes shrinking, which "shuts the wolf into the sheep-fold". This blocks the normal drainage of the poisoned lymph, and then the toxic matter has plenty of time to inflame the walls of its prison.

We use the term "cellulitis" for this disease, cellular tissues being synonymous with connective tissue.

Is cellulitis exclusive to women? No, 30% of cases afflict men. If a man pays less attention to it, it's because his trouble is less visible. It doesn't start in his legs as the women's does. Its beginnings are modestly concealed under his jacket or his belt. While cellulitis affects women in particular, they are not its only victim—far from it. It is simply that it attacks them at the prime of life and is more easily noticed by others.

THE DIAGNOSIS

Cellulitis begins on the inside surface of the thighs and knees, covering up the bone projections. It quickly moves down to thicken the ankles, which disappear from view. This thickening becomes more and more pronounced and soon affects the whole leg (which hardens) from the ankle to the knee. Gradually but relentlessly, over the months and years, the thickening of the lower limbs continues and the sides of the thighs swell out in their turn.

Then the hips become heavy with rolls of fat, as do the buttocks. From there, the process pads out the rest of the body and produces thick necks, swollen napes and heavy shoulders.

In cases of virtually generalized cellulitis, which are happily rare, the unfortunate patients find themselves imprisoned in a painful, thick and almost rigid shell which must cause them the most intense discomfort.

At first the tissues still have a soft consistency and are not painful. This is at the stage when the mucus is invading the connective tissues, and it may be difficult to distinguish from watery or fatty infiltration. You can be guided by the place where it appears. Cellulitis first shows on the inside of the thigh and knees.

Later, pinching the skin is painful and may produce small wrinkles even in the early stages. Cellulitis may also be suspected at this early stage from the badly nourished appearance of the skin which is rough, greyish and cold.

At the stage of confirmed cellulitis, the symptoms are clear:

1. When the skin is handled, it can be perceived to be *infiltrated,* giving the impression of being composed of nodules which, from their firmness and contours, give a feeling of padding.
2. The skin adheres to the underlying tissues, instead of being loosely separated from them.

In cases of cellulitis, the connective tissue between the skin and the underlying tissues, instead of making for suppleness, becomes inflamed and consequently adheres to what is above and below it. So if the skin is pinched, it will be observed that it is adhering to the deep layers by a number of small fibres which hold down the skin, forming small depressions.

3. Pinching is painful and easily causes bruising.

This phrase corresponds to the inflammation of the connective tissue through the action of the poisoned lymph which surrounds it.

At the atrophy stage, you will feel underneath the skin small balls or little grains: a kind of nodule which rolls around under your fingers.

The areas attacked by cellulitis are:

- The inside surface of the thighs.
- The knees. (Remember that fat reaches this level only at a late stage. If there is abnormal thickening just above the joint on the inside, beware).
- The ankles.
- The hips.
- The nape of the neck, causing painful thickening rising to the base of the skull and the scalp.
- The backs of the arms.

Occasionally, the shoulder-blades and spinal column.

It can sometimes appear on the forehead and the lower part of the face.

The dangers

Cellulitic overweight does not bring the organic disorders caused by obesity. You can die from obesity—you will not die of cellulitis. But because of the ill-effects it does have, treatment is sufficiently necessary for a list of its real dangers to be more than a matter of idle curiosity. You **must** know what risks you are taking in letting it develop.

You first notice the increasing unsightliness it produces: the well known monsterlike deformity. The lower limbs can assume enormous proportions where any idea of curves, knees and ankles will be but a memory.

More seriously, cellulitis will give rise to nervous pressure, resulting in severe pains, which may become terrible, like branding with a red hot poker or a feeling of being bitten. These occur more often at night, giving rise to insomnia, which contributes further to the disorder of the nervous system.

Ageing, though less serious, is of more usual concern. Faces affected by cellulitis while still young, fade rapidly although the complexion is attractive and the cheeks rounded. But this roundness is a sign of swelling rather than of healthy tissue. When this swelling of a tissue, which is really undernourished, suddenly collapses, it leaves more wrinkles than would normally be the case.

Factors favouring the onset of cellulitis

Heredity. It is difficult to decide whether cellulitis is transmitted directly or is brought on by liver or kidney defects transmitted from mother to daughter. The latter explanation seems the more plausible. In any event, it is a fact that a cellulitic mother will often have a cellulitic daughter.

Feeding: Cellulitis being a blockage of the system by poisons which it has no means of neutralizing, the importance of the quality of the food intake is obvious. I use the word quality deliberately, as quantity is no longer the most important thing here. If the patient is a large eater, she will saddle herself anyway with ordinary overweight in addition to cellulitis. But you don't have to eat a lot to get cellulitis. All you have to do is to eat in a way which runs counter to the principles of healthy living.

Cellulitis is conditioned by taking in indigestible foods—very fatty pork meats, stews, sauces, fried foods and such and alcoholic drinks. In a word: anything which first attacks the liver and having broken down its defence mechanism, brings in poison which the body cannot destroy and therefore stores hastily way in the cellular lymph.

Cellulitis, like many other diseases, is a defence reaction of the body. It is the body's way of coping with the fire. Poisonous though it be, the intruder is shut up in the room where it will cause the least disturbance, thus freeing the other organs from its harmful influence.

Resumption of the normal activity of the liver, under the influence of dieting and treatment, is vital if on the one hand the poisons in the intestine are to be rendered harmless and on the other hand normal cellular purification is to assist and consolidated the treatment.

Sedentariness. There are two ways of dealing with poisons. The first is to render them harmless chemically. This is done by the digestive tract. The second is to burn them up. We are now going to examine the inadequacy of this means of defence.

It is said nowadays that the way to burn up poisons is to exercise your muscles. Actually, what we should really say is that we have to exercise our muscles enough to produce a complete combustion of the carbons which the body sends them. Incomplete combustion begets toxins.

Let us pursue this idea, which is of importance in relation to physical and breathing exercises.

Once the poisons have crossed the barrier of the digestion and have not yet been driven into the cellular storehouses, they enjoy a short period of freedom in the general bloodstream.

At this stage, they may still be destroyed in two ways: if their concentration is not too strong, they can be disposed of by the kidneys. They can still be burnt up.

They can be burnt up only by oxygen. Oxygen can consume poisons at only two points, the lungs and the muscles. The two must work together for purification to take place.

But, note this, if the muscle is working in too confined a space, not oxygenated, it does not burn well. It causes incomplete oxidation and so itself forms poisons (lactic acid) which causes blockages and spread through the body. This is the phenomenon of fatigue.

Fatigue, like sedentariness is an important factor in cellulitis. Moderate exercise is good. Tiring oneself out is not. It is not good enough to go and shut oneself into a dance hall and sweat and then say: "Well, I keep moving". Nor is it good enough just to go about your household chores in your usual way.

All these occupations do, of course, give a change from sitting down, but you have to learn to breathe and to breathe in the open air. You must do sensible physical exercise and not over-exert yourself, more particularly since every occasion on which you put a strain on yourself (especially by staying up late) is often simply a fresh opportunity for further poisoning with food and alcohol. Sophisticated city life is a major cause of cellulitis.

It is not the task of the **kidneys** to render poisons harmless. Their job is to spot them and throw them out. This is our purification system.

If the kidneys function inadequately, they will not chase out the excess poisons. At a more advanced stage, they will even convert a body with a normal percentage of toxins into a highly poisoned body by not letting any toxins go and allowing them to become more and more concentrated in the blood. It follows that healthy kidneys are extremely important. This fact ought to be a further reason for avoiding poisonous foods such as alcohol, which is threefold factor in cellulitis. It attacks at three basic defences at once—the digestive system, the nervous system and the kidney system.

Chapter VIII

The Treatment for Cellulitis

DIETING

Judicious eating with a low calorie content. Good food should make up for the normal wear and tear on our tissues. If the work entailed in assimilating food is less than counter balanced by the benefit derived from it, one can say that running cost are exceeding income. We are in effect spending part of our reserves of vitality in neutralising the toxins which are contained in certain foods, and thus losing the overall benefit.

When we haven't enough vitality to burn up the excess poison and deal adequately with an intake which is difficult to assimilate, there must result a general fouling-up of all the bodily processes.

So we must ban everything which is highly seasoned—condiments, spices, salt and pepper or toxic-coffee, alcohol, tea, tobacco, highly fermented cheese-or too acid-tomatoes, lemons or over-cooked-stews, fatty pork meats, sauces, high game, cooked butter, fried foods, fish with highly seasoned sauces.

Here is a more detailed list of foods which the cellulitic should, avoid as much as possible:

- *Fish, salted and preserved* caviare, anchovies, sardines, cod, tunny, haddock.
- *Oily fish*: eels, mackerel, herring.
- *Certain meats*: foie gras, duck, goose, fatty pork meats, stews, guinea-fowl, game, pork, tripe.
- *Shellfish*: lobsters, crabs, crayfish, prawns, mussels, scallops.
- *Vegetables*: broad beans, split peas, soya.
- *Fruit*: all dried fruits.
- *Milk products*: strong Cheese.
- *Confectionery*: all.
- *Condiments*: all spicy things (mustard, pickles, garlic).
- *Drinks*: all alcoholic drinks, coffee and tea.
- *Tobacco*: two cigarettes a day at the most.

Thanks to this diet, which will include particularly meat grilled with a little butter and non-concentrated foods in general, the body will not be tired by difficult digestion. Such digestion would use up all the patient's energies and induce the well-known drowsiness which follows a heavy meal.

Eat meals at regular hours and do not eat between meals. Eat slowly, chewing well, and not reading.

Try hard to eat in peace, away from noise and problems. Relax completely during meals.

Many writers who confuse watery overweight with cellulitis advise for the latter the diet which is recommended for dealing with water retention: a dry diet, rich in meat, poor in vegetables and fruit. This is an unjustified extension of a rich meat diet to an illness which doesn't require it at all.

On the contrary, a cellulitic will need only a cooling diet, rich in green vegetables, and well-balanced menus. A vitamin table will enable you to apportion the various components of your meals wisely.

There is no need to limit your diet to dull meals. You can prepare some very good meals every day by following the principles of healthy eating, that is a diet rich in vegetables, with a reasonable amount of meat. You can, while following these principles, present the food in a sufficiently attractive and varied form to make up very appetising meals.

Here are the kind of menus we advise:

- **Breakfast:** coffee or tea, with milk (half and half), with bread and butter or oatmeal.
- **2 meals:**

— raw salad, unpeeled potatoes and slices of hard-boiled egg, peas, carrots, grated raw cabbage,
— a dessertspoonful of wheat-germ,
— a 1/4 lb. meat or an egg, or ham of lean fish,
— a vegetable,
— cheese or yoghurt. In the evening, more salad,
— fruit,
— a sweet dessert. In the evening, another dish with an egg,
— drinks: A little wine, no coffee after the meal. A glass of sherry once a fortnight.

No cocktails: Whisky only rarely. One cigarette after the meal.

Here is a "full" diet as an example.

De-poisoning diet (anti-cellulitis)

Breakfast will consist of one cup of coffee or weak tea, with one-third milk and a buttered rusk or oatmeal. No more tea or coffee to be taken all day.

All alcoholic drinks are forbidden, except for an occasional glass of red wine with meals.

You may eat 2 rusks during each meal.

I would underline that I am giving you here a diet designed to get rid of poisons and to dissolve cellulitis. *It is not a slimming diet.* Cellulitis does cause local and painful deformities but is rarely the sole factor in serious overweight.

You may use the following vegetables as you please according to the season, mixing three or four of them into one hors-d'oeuvre if you wish: beetroot, carrot, potato, green or black olives, celery, chicory, lettuce, chives, asparagus, onion, radish, peas, green beans, artichokes, endive, parsley, cauliflower, red cabbage.

MONDAY (1st and 3rd weeks)

- **Lunch:** raw mixed salad, 1 dessertspoonful of w h e a t g e r m 1/4lb grilled beef, steamed potato, pear.
- **Dinner:** lettuce, peas, yoghurt.

TUESDAY (1st and 3rd)

- **Lunch:** raw mixed salad, a spoonful of wheat-germ, veal, lettuce, yoghurt.
- **Dinner:** noodles with butter, asparagus, pear.

WEDNESDAY (1st and 3rd)

- **Lunch:** raw mixed salad, a spoonful of wheat-germ, whiting, spinach, apple.
- **Dinner:** lettuce, steamed potato, small cream cheese.

THURSDAY (1st and 3rd)

- **Lunch:** raw mixed salad and wheat-germ,

slice of roast lamb noodles with butter, small cream cheese.

- **Dinner:** green beans, chicory, apple.

FRIDAY (1st and 3rd)

- **Lunch:** raw mixed salad and wheat-germ, 2 fried eggs, asparagus, pineapple.
- **Dinner:** artichokes, carrots, cheese.

SATURDAY (1st and 3rd)

- **Lunch:** raw mixed salad and wheat-germ, lamb chop, beans, cottage cheese.
- **Dinner:** peas, spinach, banana.

SUNDAY (1st and 3rd)

- **Lunch:** raw mixed salad and wheat-germ, breast of chicken, chicory, ice cream.
- **Dinner:** spaghetti, lettuce, pear or grapes.

MONDAY (2nd and 4th weeks)

- **Lunch:** raw mixed salad and wheat-germ, rabbit, creamed potatoes, fresh figs or apple.
- **Dinner:** beans, chicory, cheese.

TUESDAY (2nd and 4th)

- **Lunch:** raw mixed salad and wheat-germ, ham, artichokes, cheese.
- **Dinner:** steamed potatoes, peas, apple.

WEDNESDAY (2nd and 4th)

- **Lunch:** raw mixed salad and wheat-germ, whiting, carrots, banana.
- **Dinner:** noodles, lettuce, cottage cheese.

THURSDAY (2nd and 4th)

- **Lunch:** raw mixed salad and wheat-germ, macaroni or spaghetti, lettuce, cream cheese.
- **Dinner:** artichokes, lettuce or celery, pineapple.

FRIDAY (2nd and 4th)

- **Lunch:** raw mixed salad and wheat-germ, fillets of sole, spaghetti, apples or strawberries.
- **Dinner:** asparagus, peas, apple.

SATURDAY (2nd and 4th)

- **Lunch:** raw mixed salad and wheat-germ, lamb's kidneys, peas, Swiss cheese.
- **Dinner:** carrots, noodles, fruit in season.

SUNDAY (2nd and 4th)

- **Lunch:** raw mixed salad and wheat-germ, calves, liver, spinach, peaches, apple or grapes.
- **Dinner:** antichoke, lettuce, yoghurt.

May you never break these rules and have a more elaborate meal, drinks when you have guests or when you visit friends? I would not go so far as to say that, but I must insist on one point. Cellulitics can not afford these "extras" more than twice a month. *They must be moderate.* Ask the doctor to prescribe a digestive remedy for such occasions.

Further, these rules for healthy eating will enable you to avoid *constipation,* which is a cause of cellulitis. If it does occur, all steps must be taken to overcome it. You must get into the habit of keeping to a definite time each day and, if necessary, take a light laxative.

EXERCISE

We have seen that physical exercise plays a part in burning up poisons. So if you are going to stop the body fluids becoming clogged and so make things easier for your natural means of defence, you must make sure that you exercise your muscles sufficiently.

But too violent exercise resulting in fatigue, increases the poisoning of the system and has precisely the opposite effect of what we want.

What cellulitics need is plenty of fresh air (we shall return to this) plus a sufficiently active muscular life.

The light exercise which is specially recommended for them *open-air walking.*

But, for severe cases of cellulitis we would advise the minimum of activity. A walk in the open air, at first once and then twice a day (provided this doesn't cause tiredness or pain). If you live in the country or the suburbs, the problem is easier to solve than if you live in town. But even in town you can get the necessary oxygen from this kind of exercise in the parks and gardens.

For how long should we walk? There is no single rule for everybody—each has his own staying power and resistance. *See that you never reach the limit.* Only go as far and as quickly as gives an agreeable and refreshing walk with no weariness.

The length you walk may be increased from five minutes the first day to half-an-hour after a week, three-quarters of an hour after a fortnight, half-an-hour twice a day after three weeks. And please, ladies, do not wear high heeled shoes.

It is an absolute principle that walking and breathing exercise are the only two forms of physical activity permitted to confirmed cellulitics at the beginning of their treatment.

It is only with cases of cellulitis in the very early stages, or with cases of confirmed cellulitis which have been treated for three to four months already, that one can go on to the next stage. Then and only then may you safely and advantageously add, to your walking and breathing exercises, a series of daily very gentle exercises which are really no more than auto-massage of the areas affected by thickening.

Here is a typical session, which has been worked out by my colleague and friend Robert Raynaud:

Typical session of physical training to overcome cellulitis

This is to be undertaken (by a confirmed cellulitic) *only after 4 months treatment.*

It is of course understood that exercises will not of themselves cure cellulitis. They are used merely as a complement to general treatment to increase its effectiveness and to speed up its good work, to restore the tone of the muscles and to prevent their re-thickening.

The movements must be easy at first, reaching their proper intensity only when the patient is completely or almost completely cured.

Here, by way of an example, is a simple session whose effects are directed at the customary cellulitic areas.

1. Little running steps until you are slightly out of breath.

2. Stand with arms stretched out in front of you at shoulder level and shoulder distance apart. Quickly cross your right arm over your left and than vice versa (like garden shears). Then stretch them to the sides

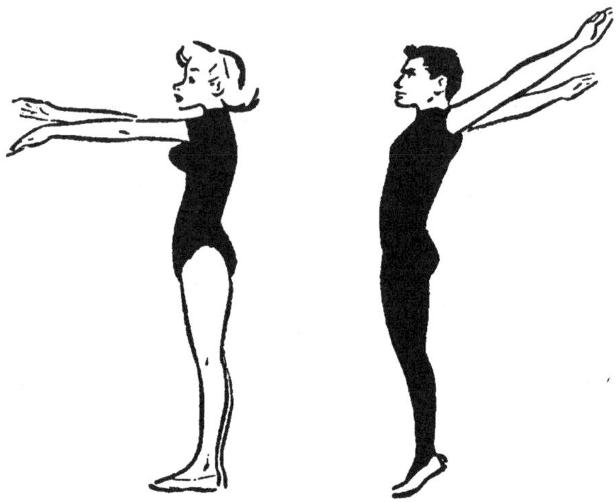

and force them as far behind you as you can 20 to 25 times.

3. Arms stretched outwards to the sides, describe two large horizontal figure of eight with your fingertips. For the forward loops the arms should approach one another in front at the level of the chin. For the backward loops, they are carried as far back as possible *20 to 30 times.*

4. Swing one outstretched arm up vertically while the other remains down behind your body. Change over, continuing without stopping at the end of each movement. *20 to 30 times.*

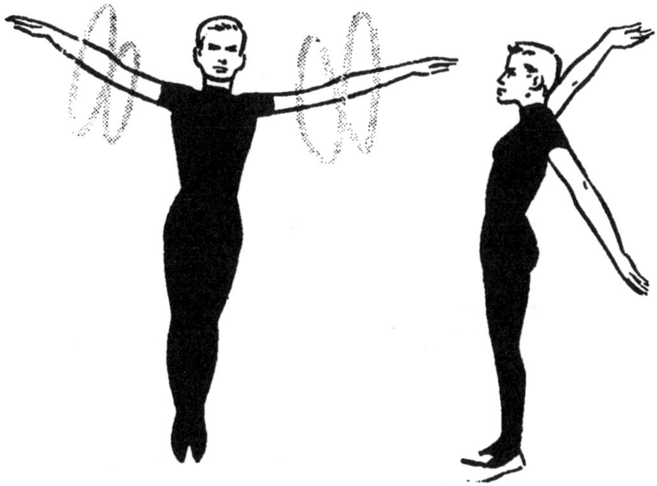

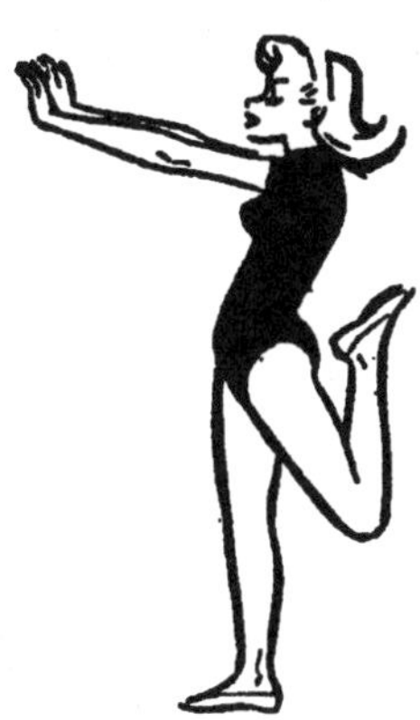

5. Strike the back of the thighs or buttocks vigorously and rapidly with the heel. Take the knee of the bent leg as far back as possible (resting the hands against a wall). *30 to 35 times each leg (see drawing).*

6. Lie flat on the stomach. Lift each leg separately to the vertical. *20 times each leg* (see drawing).

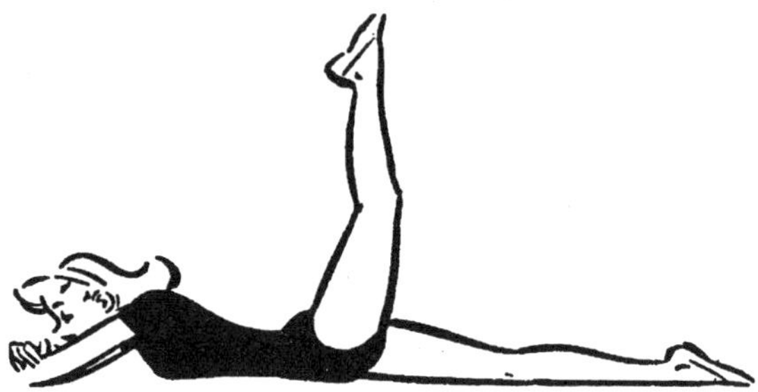

7. Stand, legs wide apart. Sit on one heel bending the leg double. While keeping the buttocks close to the ground, swing over to the other leg and sit on the opposite heel. *20 to 25 times.* (See drawing below)

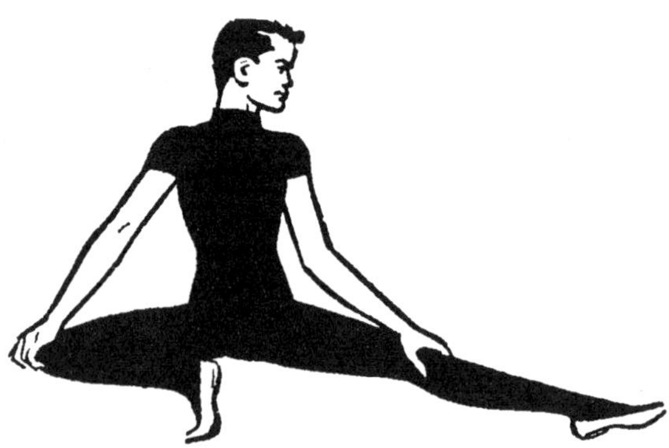

8. Kneel on the ground sitting on the heels, trunk leaning forward, arms stretched out forwards in line with the body. Swing the arms and trunk to the right in a semi-circular movement, then to the left, without stopping at the end of each movement and getting your chest down close to your knees. *20 to 25 times.* (See drawing below).

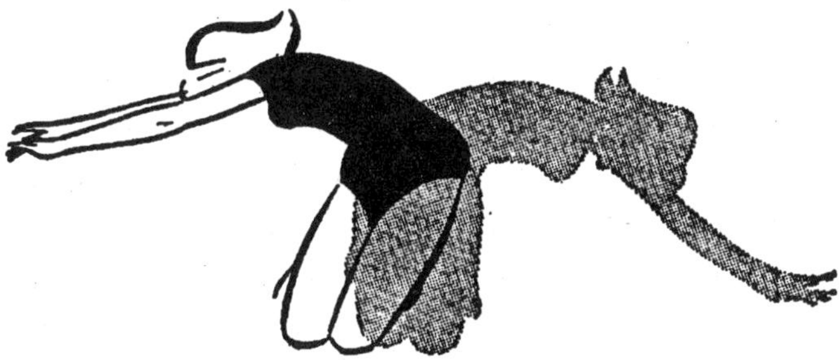

9. Lie flat on the back, arms stretched back on the floor in line with the body. Lift the legs over the head

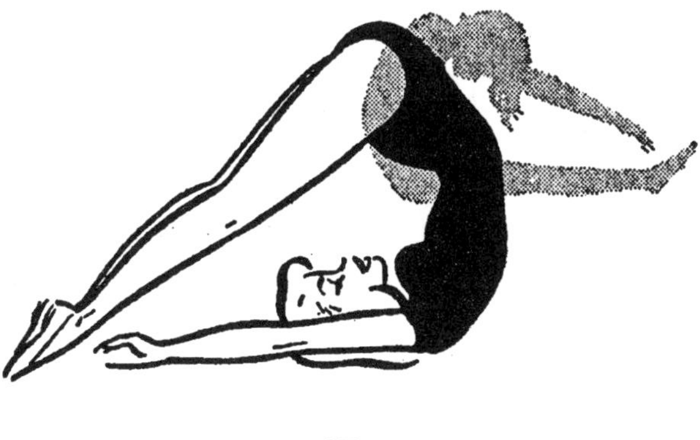

trying to touch the hands with the feet, then lower them to the floor again. *20 to 25 times.* (See drawing as shown on previous page).

- You should do these exercises as soon as you get out of bed in the morning, with the windows open (half-open in cold weather), wearing shorts and a woollen pullover. They should be followed by a high-pressure cold shower and a general alcohol rub.

Of course these exercises, whose purpose is to thin down the crucial points of cellulitic thickening, namely the hips, waist, stomach and lower limbs, must be carried out with *great discretion.* We repeat that they can be dangerous unless they are done with care. *They should not produce any aches or pains. If they do, they are harmful* and must be stopped at once. The patient should then go back to walking and gentle breathing exercises.

REST

It is not only immoderate physical exercise that causes strain. Everyday life, life pure and simple, the harassed life which is the lot of most town dwellers, causes it too. The body substance and nerve centres have to be restored at regular intervals, just as accumulators have to be recharged. Like vegetables and the lower animals, we too are subject to the great law of periodic rest.

We must learn how to rest whenever we can. Even if it is only for a quarter of an hour, between two jobs, in an armchair, with our feet up, in the shade, in silence, forcing ourselves to relax and to think of nothing.

These breaks are still more valuable before and after meals. This is the secret of many people whose tirelessness we admire—these moments of relaxation.

What we must do is to take refuge from the distractions and excitements which wear down the majority of our fellow men. The restlessness of modern life, with the telephone, traffic, the noise and the struggle to earn a living, isn't enough for them. They have to add yet other commitments, private and public. The result is more meeting to be squeezed in by fighting against the clock, or late night eating and drinking sessions.

You must learn to make your choice. If your working life is already exhausting, don't add to it the unnecessary strain of numerous nights out. If you do, you won't last and, to stick to our subject, cellulitis will catch up on you.

Here again, everyone must decide for himself what he needs. Generally speaking, 8½ hours' sleep is essential for people who use up a lot of energy. The ideal is to go to bed at 10.30 and get up at 7 a.m. Only one weekly outing or party which keeps you up till 1 o'clock in the morning—not more.

Take you annual vacation when the weather is warm. Holidays are not a luxury. We don't need to point that out.

For human beings, as for all living things, animal and vegetable, winter should be period of comparative rest, when life slows down and the body quietly awaits the awakening of spring. *So avoid overdoing winter sports.* Yes, go to the mountains in winter. The air there is splendid for you. But don't put on skis unless you habitually indulge in sport throughout the year, and in that case you would not have cellulitis. But, if you have got it, forget about the skis. Look at the mountains, fill your lungs with pure fresh air, dress warmly, and stroll about in the snow and sunshine. That alone will make the trip worthwhile.

In short, learn how to rest. Learn not to waste your energies, and you will already be on the road to health, which is the road to happiness.

BREATHING

I have already stressed the important part played by breathing in burning up the poisons in the blood. Oxygen is the great purifier to the bloodstream, but our lungs need something else from the air. They want all the vital forces in the atmosphere which come from the sun, from the earth and are breathed out by every living thing—flowers, birds, trees and men. You must surely have noticed that the presence of some people cheers you up while that of others depresses you, as if we were all vitality accumulators and as if the diversity of our respective potentials caused current to flow between us.

We must find fresh air. We must shun stuffy atmospheres and crowded streets, as much because of our need for oxygen as because of our need for this vital force. On roads, where exhaust fumes and factory smoke hang about and where you are bombarded by the air breathed by the crowd, you will hardly find either.

At least try to make the most of the available air by learning how to breath. Few people know how to do this. Few know how to turn to advantage this marvellous means of increasing the bodily capacity and life potential. Every morning, before doing your physical exercises (if you are allowed to do them) practise a series of complete breathing exercises which will take the purifying oxygen into your innermost being. In this way, breathing will become one of your most effective weapons in the fight against cellulitis.

In order to achieve a fuller airing of your lungs,

you must first understand the basic mechanism of breathing. We breathe:

- By inflating the stomach (abdominal breathing).
- By dilating the chest (thoracic breathing).

This abdominal breathing consists of lowering the muscles of the diaphragm which is the partition separating the chest from the abdomen. It can easily be seen that this lowering diminishes the capacity of the abdomen as compared with that of the thorax and swells the stomach, by compressing the intestines, giving the lungs more room for expansion.

Women rarely breathe using the stomach. They breathe only with the chest, and frequently only with the upper part of it. It is essential that, when doing complete breathing exercises, you breathe with the whole of your chest and with your stomach.

Do these exercises *standing up,* so that the diaphragm has free movement, ensuring that the expansion of the thorax is not hindered in any way.

In that position, start **breathing in** gently, first inflating the upper part of the thorax, and moving the arms to the horizontal and then slightly backwards. Continue to breathe in with the shoulders well back. Don't stop breathing in until your stomach is fully distended. The complete breathing-in process in all its successive stages, should take 6 seconds, and 12 seconds when you are in trim.

Breathing out, which should be done slowly. Begin by collapsing the upper part of the chest, then the lower part, and end by contacting the stomach. At the same time lower the arms, the shoulders and the head being bent slightly forward, the back slightly arched, so as to empty the chest completely. Breathing out should last almost as long as breathing in.

These movements should be done for at least three minutes, three times a day, but you can do them for longer if you wish. When you are more in trim, you can make the following variation: do the exercise *kneeling*, with your hands clasped behind the nape of your neck. When breathing out, sit on your heels lean forward till your forehead is touching your knees, hands still clasped behind your neck.

The ideal is to do these exercises while walking in the open air, holding the breath for 4 to 5 second before breathing out.

Knowing how to breathe is one of the most valuable secrets of beauty, of health and vitality. It helps to rid the system of poisons, and the cellulitis will recede. It is then and then only that you can do physical exercises as such, always doing all the breathing exercises first.

Massage

Sensible feeding, rest and proper breathing, which are imperative for a healthy life, are the vital prerequisites for the cure of cellulitis. They can prevent it, but cannot cure it alone. This is a job for careful massage.

Gentle and gradually increasing massage, which arouses sensation rather than pain, will always dispel cellulitis from the place to which it is applied, and may even cause it to disappear from areas which haven't yet been treated.

MASSAGING YOURSELF

It is often difficult, owing to lack of time perhaps, to go to a masseur for treatment. It would then be useful for your to know how to do the movements yourself, and do them well.

THE PRINCIPLES OF MASSAGE

We have already explained how you can detect the affected areas yourself. The intensity of the inflammation can be measured by the degree of pain felt when the skin is pinched.

When you have located the cellulitic areas and duly classified them according to their degree of infiltration, first massage the whole body with a stroking and then a smoothing action very lightly and quickly, then concentrate your time and attention on the most painful area and on that only (see p. 105).

This massage should never cause you pain, but should be hard enough all the same to arouse more sensitivity than it would have done on a perfectly healthy area.

You will notice:

- That with the same amount of sensitivity but without ever causing pain, the massage in the same place will get deeper and deeper and more and more energetic. You will then move on to the other areas, again working gently to begin with.
- That these massages, far from leaving a bruised feeling, will rather produce a sensation of relaxation and well-being.
- That after about ten sessions the areas treated will improve spectacularly.
- That areas not yet treated will also diminish solely from the soothing and relaxing effect which the massage has brought to the irritated state of the sympathetic system which, pacified, has relaxed its hold and drawn in its claws. To put it less picutresquely, the massage has increased the flow of blood and lymph, thereby improving the circulation.

THE TECHNIQUE OF MASSAGE

Draining movements

The first is stroking (see drawing); this must be done lightly and slowly, without talc, and only with

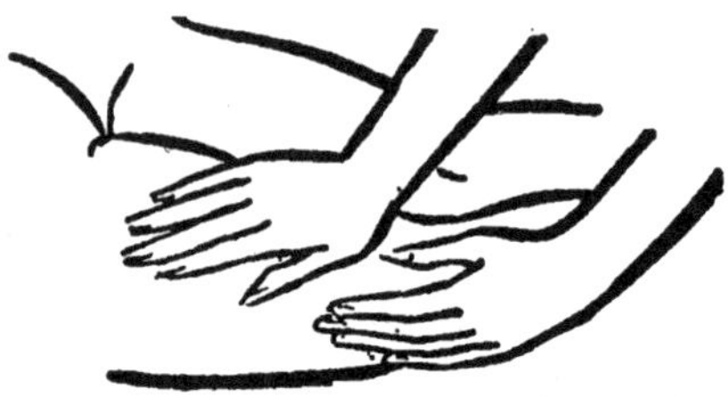

the tips of the fingers. It acts as a sedative and, if done by someone else, induces a blissful drowsiness. If the massage were sharp and quick it would increase the cellular spasms and would cause an undesirable retraction of the flesh.

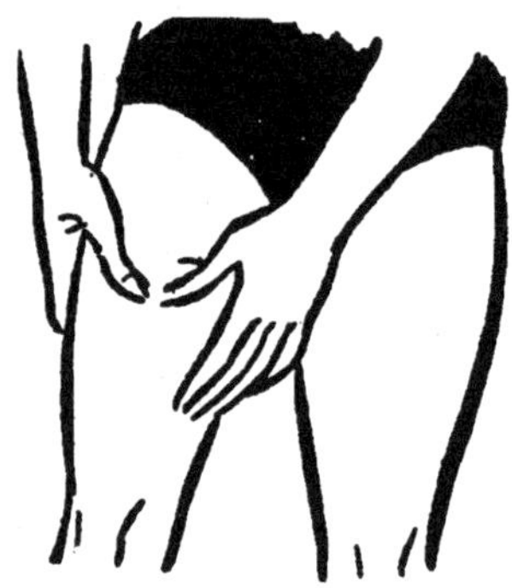

• **The second is smoothing** which is done with talc, with the palm of the hand. It goes deeper than the stroking and must always come after the latter to obey the rule of gradual increase. The hands try to mould the muscle contours and to smooth over them without grasping them, just as you would apply sunburn lotion to your skin.

These two movements are essential introductions to each massage session. They should also complete it. They have a sedative and anaesthetic influence, but especially they prepare the way for the evacuation of serous liquid which *kneading* will release. They will, in effect, clear the large "drains", preparing them to receive the lymphatic flow set in motion by the unblocking. That's why we have called them "draining movements," by analogy with the terms used in homeopathy.

This, then, is what you must do:

- **For the limbs.** Always massage *from the extremities* and especially on the inside surfaces. Pay particular attention to the hollows behind the knees and the bends of the elbows where there are the first important ganglion centres. You can rub each leg upwards with both hands at once, grasping the limb between them, or you can use each hand in turn. You will however use only one hand for each arm, lifting it up so as to be able to get hold of the inside with the other hand more easily.
- **For the stomach.** Use your right hand for anticlockwise circular massage starting at the centre and working outwards.
- **For the main lymphatic centres just below the surface.** *From the groin,* make a movement with each hand up the inside of the thigh, follow the fold of the groin and move sideways up to the base of the chest.

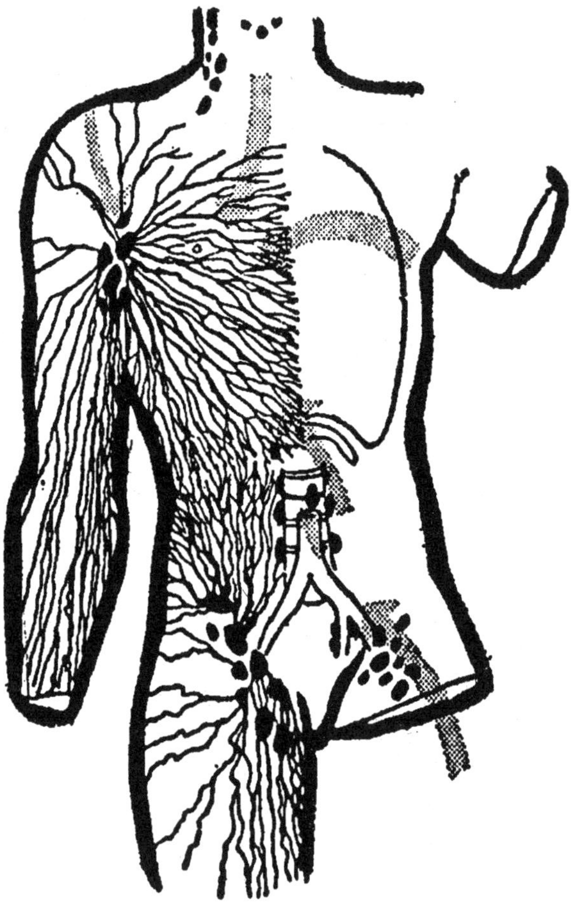

For the cellular tissue of the neck in front and behind, make fanning movements, always working downwards.

To help to free lymphatic blockage *in the armpits,* make a wide movement with the other hand, starting from the inside of the arm, over the surface of the armpit and ending below the breast.

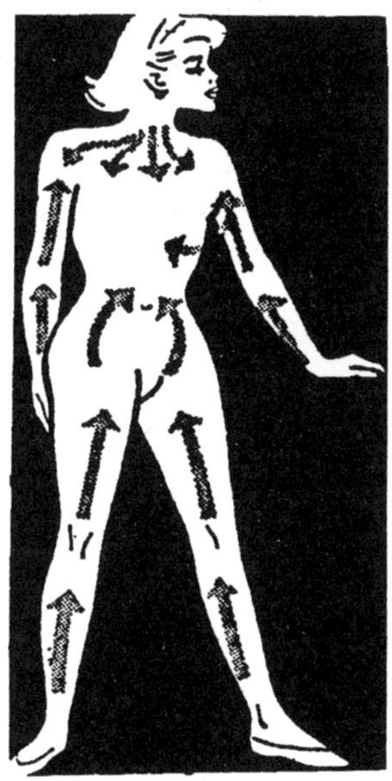

• **To sum up:** the stroking, and the smoothing action which follows it and for which it is merely a preparation, are the two drainage movements which must precede and follow massage and which must be done in the direction of the lymphatic flow (See page 108).

Kneading movements

Here are Wetterwald's three movements. The basic movement, which is at the root of all of them, consists of taking hold as generously as you can of a large fold of skin with both hands.

Direction of stroking thumbs forward, your hands 1 in. to 1½ in. apart.

• **Breadcrumb movement.** You roll this fold, rubbing the pads of the fingers across it one against the other as if you were crumbling bread.

When the skin becomes less painful, take it in both hands, still keeping the fold well in it. This is the kneading. It is the main movement in massage and is actually only an enlargement of the breadcrumb movement.

• **The two S movement.** Before letting go of this fold, make it suddenly into an S-shape by lowering one of the two parts of the fold in relation to the other. Then, equally suddenly, lower the other one, to make another S but reversed.

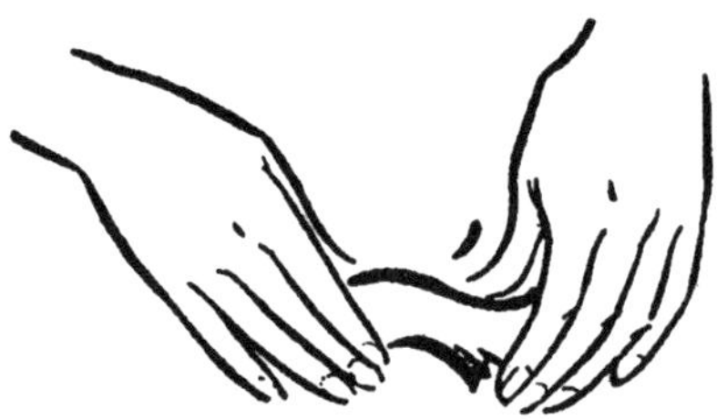

• **Wave movement.** When you have finished this movement, still do not let go of the skin but keep making the 1 to 1½ in. folds by a wave movement or like the spreading ripple on a pond. When you have reached this stage, stop there and repeat the two previous movements (the breadcrumb and the two S).

It is obvious that the two S movement, which needs both hands, cannot be done to the arms or to any other area which can be reached by only one hand. You will have to be content with the breadcrumb movement, moving it along 1½ in. at a time by the wave movement.

In any event never cover more than about 6 in. at one session.

First aid movements

- **Flat-pressure movement.** It may be impossible to do Wetterwald's movements because the skin is adhering and absolutely refuses to allow itself to be folded. This is often so with the backs and outside of the thighs. Then you have to use the *flat-pressure movement* to make the Wetterwald movements possible later. This consists of pulling apart the areas which are adhering with the palms of both hands placed flat an inch or so apart. Use a circular movement so as to free the surface tissues as much as possible, then try to bring the palms together to create a fold between them.

In due course this movement will give a certain suppleness to the surface areas and will enable them to slide lightly over the lower levels. As soon as you have got a sufficient fold on the outside skin to be able to apply the Wetterwald movements, change to them.

• **Finger kneading.** Flat-pressure is possible only if you can press down on a solid lower plane. When this is impossible, as for instance in the case of the stomach, you loosen up the skin with the pads of your fingers, the hands facing one another and at an angle of 35 deg. to the skin.

These then are 5 main kneading movements:

— the 3 Wetterwald movements: the breadcrumb (extended later to become kneading), the two S and the wave,

— the 2 complementary movements: flat-pressure and finger kneading.

You will decide for yourself which movement best suits the area you want to treat. This will be the one which produces sufficient feeling while never becoming painful and which when finished will leave only a sensation of relaxation and well-being. You must always do the movement as deeply and energetically as possible, while keeping strictly within the limits of this basic rule: you must never experience a feeling of bruising.

These movements must never be done on a "dry" skin. Use talc or better still a decongestive and analgesic cream. There are several suitable creams on the market.

The massage timetable

The best time for massage is in the morning, when the inflammation of the cellulitic tissue is at its minimum.

Cellulitics is always more evident in the evening because of fatigue. Conversely, the tissues are relatively deflated in the morning because the body has rested and has been in a horizontal position, which always helps the elimination of organic liquids.

Morning massage can be deeper, hence more effective. Incipient cellulitis should also be massaged in the morning, even if it is in fact not apparent at the beginning of the day. All you need to do is to note, the previous evening, which areas require treatment.

Do the massage three times a week, 35 minutes each time.

Draining: 5 minutes

Roll-massage: 5 minutes

Rapid superficial attack on all the least affected areas: 10 minutes.

Direct attack on the most painful areas: 10 minutes.

General draining movements: 5 minutes.

Finish with a cold shower and friction with a loofah or rough towel.

You will be able to recognize good and effective massage by the fact that the ganglions (of the groins for the legs, of the armpits for the arms) have enlarged and do not hurt after the session. If the massage is too violent, the ganglions will not enlarge until the next day and will be painful.

OTHER TREATMENTS

- mention, merely for reference, expressotherapy by compressed-air or by pneumatic bandages which are undoubtedly effective.
- should like to lay further stress on:
- **The Danish traxador method** of massage by a aspiration, which is used by most large thermal institutions.

Instead of working on the skin, the connective tissue and the muscles by manual kneading, they are sucked up by the vacuum formed by a sort of "bell-glasses" of various sizes according to the part of the body being treated. This sets up a moving wave, full of lymph, which is made to travel in the same direction as the lymphatic circulation. This produces an artificial lymphatic current whose movement frees and sweeps away the static toxins in the subcutaneous cellular tissue. All this is done painlessly.

- **The kinesitherapeutic roller.** The kine-roller is an electrically-operated roller. The stroking roll is made of ultrasmooth plastic cylinders mounted on flexible axles and makes use of the clever idea of oblique sweeping done by the road-sweeping vehicles. The intention is to produce a hollowness similar to that of the hand and its aims and results are as good as the traxator. In the kneading roll, designed to deal with old-established and fibrous cellulitis, there are rows of wooden balls instead of the plastic tubes.

DRUGS FOR CELLULITIS

There are of course all the drugs which work indirectly through their beneficial action on the liver or kidneys to reinforce the anti-poison defences of our body. There are also other drugs which work indirectly through their action on the nerves and the sympathetic system.

But especially to be recommended are "cures" which dispel the poisons by spa waters which ensure thorough cleansing of the blood. Your doctor will advise you of these spas which offer the appropriate cure.

Remember then that it is cellulitis if:

- It is localized. It is in definite areas and begins on the inside surface of the thighs and knees.
- The skin is infiltrated, padded and has the elastic consistency of a sheet of rubber.
- The skin is not mobile, it cannot be squeezed, and develops the "orange peel" look.
- The skin hurts when touched.
- Bruises appear very easily.

What can you do about it?

- Take regular, well-balanced meals with a low calorie content.
- Take daily exercise, prolonged but not too energetic (open-air walking, light sports).
- Rest as often as possible; relax.
- Breathe efficiently, with your chest and with your stomach.
- Massage yourself on the right principles, that is to say thoroughly but without causing pain or discomfort.

- Increase the intensity of the massage progressively, but never let it become painful.
- Before and after the proper massage, do the drainage movements (stroking and smoothing actions) in the direction of the lymphatic circulation so as to "open it up."
- Do the Wetterwald kneading movements: the breadcrumb movement (which gradually changes to kneading), the two S movements and the wave movement. These movements must always leave a feeling of relaxation and well being.
- If the latter are not possible, try "flat-pressure" and "finger kneading" by way of preparation for them.

What you must never do

- Do intensive physical exercises which require excessive effort, or practise over-violent sports.
- Start massaging vigorously right away, thereby causing discomfort.
- Get bruises after a massage.
- Get tired and stiff after walking.

- Eat indigestible foods, drink alcoholic drinks, smoke, drink too much coffee, live in a stuffy atmosphere, stay up late, wear yourself out, exhaust your nerves, work yourself up unnecessarily.
- Regularly attend badly-ventilated and smoky public places.

*Ideal Weights and Measurements for a Women**

These weights and measurements are only intended as a guide and should not be regarded as a standard. They are based on a young woman of average build. Variations in age, bone structure and muscle can affect these figures considerably.

Height	Weight	Bust	Waist	Hips
5′	116 lb.	32″	22″	34″
5′ 1″	120″	33″	23″	34″
5′ 2″	124″	33½″	23½″	34½″
5′ 3″	126″	34″	24″	35″
5′ 4″	128″	34½″	24″	36″
5′ 5″	130″	35″	24½″	37″
5′ 6″	135″	35½″	25″	37½″
5′ 7″	140″	36″	25½″	38″
5′ 8″	142″	36½″	26″	38½″
5′ 9″	145″	37″	27″	39″
5′ 10″	148″	37½″	27½″	39½″
5′ 11″	152″	38″	28″	40″

Height	Thigh	Calf	Ankle
5′	19″	11½″	6½″
5′ 1″	19½″	11½″	6½″
5′ 2″	20″	12″	7″
5′ 3″	20½″	12″	7″
5′ 4″	21″	12½″	7½″
5′ 5″	21½″	12½″	7½″
5′ 6″	22″	13″	7½″
5′ 7″	22″	13″	8″
5′ 8″	22½″	13½″	8″
5′ 9″	23″	13½″	8″
5′ 10″	23″	14″	8½″
5′ 11″	23½″	14″	8½″